Equity and Healthcare Reform in Developing Economies

Ensuring equity in healthcare is the main concern of health policymakers in order to provide a sustainable health system. This concern is more prominent in developing countries due to the scarcity of resources. This book provides a comprehensive analysis and discussion on the distributive pattern of out-of-pocket pharmaceutical expenditures under the health reforms in Turkey and makes comparisons with pharmerging countries.

Turkey's health reforms began in 2003 to address shortcomings related to financial protection and to improve health outcomes and the quality of healthcare services. The primary motivation was to ensure equity in the distribution of health resources, and this transformation process led to profound changes in how these resources were used, and in health financing in general. However, there is a lack of knowledge regarding the long-term effect of health reforms on the distribution patterns of health expenditures and health service use. This book offers a thorough equity analysis of the health financing system, affected by this health transformation program. Index and curve approaches are used in the equity analysis of pharmaceutical expenditures. The book examines the long-term effects of health system regulations on the health spending characteristics of households and improves the current understanding of equity in this context. It includes extensive international comparisons of healthcare services across a range of developing countries and highlights the significance of ensuring equity for emerging economies.

The author explores the existing evidence as well as future research directions and provides policy and planning advice for health policymakers to contribute to establishing a more equal health system design. Additionally, the book will be of interest to scholars and professionals in the fields of health economics, public health management and health financing.

Songül Çınaroğlu is a Doctor in Health Administration and Assistant Professor in the Faculty of Economics and Administrative Sciences in the Department of Health Care Management at Hacettepe University, Turkey. She is a former visiting researcher at the University of Michigan (Ann Arbor) and of the University of Alabama (Birmingham). Her main research interest is health economics, policy and outcomes research.

Routledge International Studies in Health Economics
Edited by **Charles Normand**, *Trinity College Dublin, Ireland* and
Richard M. Scheffler, *School of Public Health, University of California, Berkeley, USA*

Equity and Healthcare Reform in Developing Economies

The Case of Turkey

Songül Çınaroğlu

Routledge
Taylor & Francis Group

LONDON AND NEW YORK

First published 2021
by Routledge
2 Park Square, Milton Park, Abingdon, Oxon OX14 4RN

and by Routledge
605 Third Avenue, New York, NY 10017

First issued in paperback 2022

Routledge is an imprint of the Taylor & Francis Group, an informa business

British Library Cataloguing-in-Publication Data
A catalogue record for this book is available from the British Library

Library of Congress Cataloging-in-Publication Data
Names: Çınaroğlu, Songül, author.
Title: Equity and healthcare reform in developing economies:
the case of Turkey / Songül Çınaroğlu.
Description: Abingdon, Oxon; New York, NY: Routledge, 2021. |
Series: Routledge studies in health economics |
Includes bibliographical references and index.
Identifiers: LCCN 2020027308 (print) | LCCN 2020027309 (ebook) |
ISBN 9780367559885 (hardback) | ISBN 9781003095989 (ebook)
Subjects: LCSH: Medical care, Cost of–Turkey. | Public health–Turkey.
Classification: LCC RA410.9.T9 C56 2021 (print) |
LCC RA410.9.T9 (ebook) | DDC 362.1/042509561–dc23
LC record available at https://lccn.loc.gov/2020027308
LC ebook record available at https://lccn.loc.gov/2020027309

ISBN: 978-0-367-55990-8 (pbk)
ISBN: 978-0-367-55988-5 (hbk)
ISBN: 978-1-003-09598-9 (ebk)

DOI: 10.4324/9781003095989

Typeset in Sabon
by Newgen Publishing UK

Contents

Illustrations

Figures

Tables

Chapter 1

Equity in healthcare services

Healthcare is one of the essential policymaking sectors of the government in any country (Purnell et al., 2016). Financial resource constraints, increasing needs and expectations of health consumers, and high competition in health market necessitates considering "equity" in healthcare (Hall and Jacobson, 2018). Ensuring equity in the distribution of health resources is crucial for ensuring health system sustainability (Baum and Fisher, 2010). Lack of awareness of health policymakers regarding the health expenses of households, in areas with high cost, such as on pharmaceutical products, can affect the financially weaker sections of the society (Gemmill et al., 2008). Thus, health policymakers need to be aware of the importance of equity and should consider income-level differences when healthcare services are distributed (Khaled et al., 2018). Turkey is a developing country wherein the greatest proportion of healthcare expenditures come from public resources (Acemoglu and Ucer, 2015). As in most of the countries in the Organization for Economic Co-operation and Development (OECD), one of the primary out-of-pocket (OOP) healthcare expenditures in Turkey is medicine, and public and private expenditure on pharmaceuticals is high (Yardim et al., 2014; Ozgen-Narci et al., 2015)

After 2001, the Turkish government was able to promote stabilization as a result of reform in the public sector, and money was allocated to facilitate the increase in expenditure on healthcare and education and to improve socially inclusive growth (World Bank, 2014). Turkey's Health Transformation Program (HTP) began in 2003 and has continued since then under the auspices of the Adalet ve Kalkınma Partisi (Justice and Development Party). This program is comprehensive and includes structural reforms in the areas of organization and financing of healthcare services.

Public healthcare expenditures in Turkey have increased, especially from 2003 to 2008. This increase coincided with the establishment of the HTP and a period of sustained economic growth, followed by increased public sector investment (Atun et al., 2013; Yardim et al., 2014). During this period, members of poor households were much less likely to seek healthcare than those of nonpoor households because of concerns regarding affordability

(Brown et al., 2014). Before HTP, Turkey had a fragmented structure in the health insurance market. In 2006, as part of the unification of the health financing system, the General Health Insurance Law unified the five health insurance funds within the Sosyal Güvenlik Kurumu (Social Insurance Institution); (Akdağ, 2003). Moreover, all public hospitals formerly owned by social security funds came under the jurisdiction of the Ministry of Health.

The unification of the health financing system, including the Green Card scheme, to protect poor populations is a significant component of this reorganization process to decrease poverty and address consumer expectations. Clearly, the success of healthcare transition programs depends on incorporating patient expectations into the system and considering demographic and welfare state indicators (Meng et al., 2015). The degree of satisfaction with the healthcare services in Turkey increased from 39% in 2003 to 72.3% in 2015 (Ministry of Health, 2015). The Turkish populace view healthcare as the government's most developed policy area (Agartan, 2015), and the successful healthcare reforms reflect the popularity of the Adalet ve Kalkınma Partisi (Onis, 2015). Despite the fact that healthcare is a dynamic area of research and pharmaceutical expenditures are costly, the distributional analysis of pharmaceutical expenditures in Turkey has not been analyzed extensively. To fill this void, we analyze the level of progressivity in the distribution of pharmaceutical expenditures, using Turkey as a case study.

The objective of this chapter is to provide a closer look at the meaning of equity and health system differences regarding the consideration of equity in the light of health trends and socially inclusive policies. Therefore, in this chapter, the meaning of equity is explained first. After that, globalization and the increasing concern to ensure equity is explained. Next, healthcare system differences are indicated according to the level of primary concern to ensure equity in healthcare. Subsequently, the interrelationships between health trends and socially inclusive policies in health with equity are examined.

The meaning and key concepts of equity in healthcare

Equity has always been the primary concern for health policymakers (Purnell et al., 2016), and the primary goal in developing inclusive and equitable health policies (Atun et al., 2016). Despite the existence of significant differences in the definitions, measurements, interpretations, and determinants of equity, this issue should be the principal aim of every healthcare system (Liu et al., 2002). Health inequity is defined as the differences in health among groups of people who are avoidable, unfair, and unjust (Whitehead, 1992). Equity is characterized by social justice and fairness, and it is an ethical concept based on principles of distributive justice (Beauchamp and Childress, 1994). Equity in health can be defined as the absence of unjust and unfair health disparities in a society (Braveman and Gruskin, 2003). The terms "equality" and "equity" are often used interchangeably; however, they are different concepts. Health equity focuses on the distribution of resources and other processes. Not all disparities are unfair (Anand, 2002; Evans et al., 2001); for example, young adults in general are expected to be healthier than elderly people. Moreover, newborn girls tend to have lower birth weights on average than newborn boys (Braveman and Gruskin, 2003).

Differences in nutrition and immunizations coverage, racial/ethnic differences, and income disparities are the primary focus areas of equity research (Fiscella et al., 2000). Equity in health means that all people have an equal opportunity to be healthy. This is accomplished by the distribution and design of healthcare resources and programs, many of which are shaping and transforming the healthcare sector (Braveman and Gruskin, 2003). Indicators of health equity that have been described in the literature include education, economic status, place of residence (rural and urban), and child's sex (where applicable) (Hosseinpoor et al., 2015). Additionally, equity analysis can be applied in several contexts, such as health outcomes, specific diseases, malnutrition, maternal care, newborn and child health, accessibility of care, utilizations of healthcare services, delivery of healthcare services, financing of healthcare, insurance coverage, operations of healthcare services, and distribution of healthcare technologies (WHO, 2013a).

In this regard, equity is a multidisciplinary concept and closely related to poverty issues. Poverty is a dynamic phenomenon, and poverty-alleviation strategies have been on top of the agenda of policymakers and practitioners in healthcare (Atun et al., 2016; Deaton, 2003). Closing the gaps in healthcare disparities, interventions, and research are the primary motivations in achieving health equity (Purnell et al., 2016) and ensuring health system sustainability. In addition, globalization has created increasing economic inequality and uncertainty, which has led to a major debate on the sustainability of healthcare financing (Liaropoulos and Goranitis, 2015).

Core distributional concern in most health systems is to achieve egalitarian goals and ensure that the equity standards are met and equal treatment is provided. However, it is difficult to specify the distribution of relational egalitarian ideals of healthcare and examine what policies would best implement them (van Doorslaer et al., 1992). Egalitarians with a specific interest in health are the primary links between health; health-relevant factors; socially relevant factors; and the distribution of healthcare, public health programs, and health research (van Doorslaer et al., 1992). The motivation behind egalitarianism is to promote equal standards and establish equal standing of people to cut across different dimensions of well-being (Moss, 2007). Developing a strong economy and implementing poverty-alleviation strategies are necessary to fight against poverty. Because of the existence of a close relationship between economy and health systems, an effective health system is essential for developing a strong economy (Leach-Kemon et al.,

2012). Pursuing equity in healthcare means alleviating disparities between poor and wealthy people through government action in favor of the poor (Smith and Weinstock, 2019). Continuous monitoring of the level of equity in healthcare provides an opportunity for further policy advocacy at the national and regional levels (Bambas Nolen et al., 2005)

Moreover, simultaneous poverty-alleviation strategies supported by effective health and economic policies have helped in reducing poverty and improving health status (Atun et al., 2016). The primary objective of these policies is ensuring healthcare services for everyone (Evans et al., 2013). One of the elements of these policies is insurance coverage enhancement for citizens. However, improving medical care services and establishing affordable healthcare for the financially weaker population are the main strategies of improving the quality of healthcare systems (Levey et al., 2012). Today, under the effect of increasing chronic diseases, the OOP health expenditure, which refers to the payments made at the point of health services (Terrelonge, 2014), has increased in several countries. Additionally, pharmaceutical expenditure constitutes a significant part of OOP health expenditure (Xu et al., 2003).

The healthcare reforms that took place during the past decade to achieve equity in healthcare have led to an improvement in health outcomes and helped in creating an equitable financing system (Wagstaff, 2002). HTPs have been implemented to control and reduce OOP (Piroozi et al., 2017). Moreover, government investments and income distribution are two well-known critical factors in the health reforms that help reduce the share of OOP in total health expenditure and disposable personal income (WHO, 2013).

The principal concern of health policymakers is to devise policies to extend insurance coverage of vulnerable people so that they have continued access to healthcare services. The primary reason for the increased interest in medical insurance is to make it an incentivizing factor and to help improve the health status (Atun et al., 2016). Even though ensuring equity is the main motivation of health policymakers, every health system has its own dynamics. Therefore, it is necessary to consider globalization and personalized medicine dynamics to better understand health system differences and equity in the health system.

Globalization, personalized medicines, and an increasing concern for equity in healthcare

The progressive integration of national economies into the world economy, which is known as "globalizations," has changed the way of thinking in healthcare policymaking (Ottersen et al., 2014). Increasing evidence has shown that health inequalities exist between and within countries, and emphasis has been placed on eliminating global health inequalities (Cash-Gibson et al., 2018). Policymakers, donors, and nongovernmental

organizations are increasingly concerned about equity in healthcare for several reasons. Increased demand is one reason; in the 1980s, governments
preferred to use cost containment and efficiency to promote equity in health.
The reason for this preference was the belief that "inequalities" are ideologic-
ally unacceptable (O'Donnell et al., 2008). Researchers further familiarized
themselves with the concept of equity in the 1990s. The number of policies
and programs related to health equity increased during that decade (Evans
et al., 2001). Other reasons for the increasing popularity of equity research
in healthcare are as follows: household datasets are available and comparable for developed and developing countries; national governments are
continuously monitoring international comparability of household surveys
and are increasing the availability of data for researchers; and the use of
computers is expanding. After the introduction of personal computers at
the end of the 1980s, analysis of household datasets became easy, quick, and
cheaper. Increase in usage of analytic techniques to quantify health inequalities is another reason for the increasing interest in analysis of equity in
healthcare (van Doorslaer et al., 2004; Wagstaff and van Doorslaer, 2000).

Health equity is a priority in the post-2015 sustainable development
agenda and other major health initiatives. The World Health Organization
(WHO) has a long history of actions to achieve equity in health, including
efforts to encourage monitoring and curtailing of health inequalities. In
1948, the WHO endorsed health as a right for all, regardless of age, race,
religion, and political opinion. The WHO prioritizes the improvement of
the health status of vulnerable groups. In 1978, the *Declaration of Alma-
Ata,* advocating action to improve the health of all the people of the world,
emphasized the need to reduce inequalities within and between countries (WHO, 1978; WHO Social Determinants of Health, 2015). In 1981,
the Global Strategy for Health for All was adopted by the World Health
Assembly. In the report of this strategy, the WHO (1981) stated that the
achievement of equity depended on how healthcare resources are distributed.
Recently, the Commission on Social Determinants of Health (CSDH) was
established by the WHO to promote global movement to achieve health
equity (CSDH, 2008).

In view of the emerging post-2015 sustainable development goals (SDGs),
the importance of equity is gaining attention as a cross-cutting theme for
all development-related spheres, including health (SDGs, 2014). CSDH
provides evidence to inform effective action and to indicate "avoidable"
health inequalities (Graham, 2004). CSDH's approach focuses on the Social
Determinants of Health (SDH) perspective (WHO, 2016). The WHO offers
a broad, multidimensional definition of these determinants, describing them
as "the conditions in which people are born, grow, live, work, and age"
(SDH, 2008). Although these determinants have no consensus operational
definition, health inequalities are presumably related to income level, educational attainment, employment status, and neighborhood socioeconomic

factors (Doyle et al., 2019). These factors are well-known determinants of early childhood and schooling achievement, employment and working conditions, gender inequity, and the quality of the natural environment (WHO, 2013a). To overcome global health inequities, CSDH put forward compelling evidence based on a vast body of research. Social factors, which can be changed and controlled by policy, are largely responsible for the differences in the health outcomes in different populations and groups (WHO, 2013a).

Health is significantly determined by socioeconomic factors. Global income inequalities create inequities and lead to poor health outcomes; therefore, reducing income inequality will improve population health and well-being (Pickett and Wilkinson, 2015). According to early reviews of health inequities, health in general tends to be worse in societies with greater income inequalities (Lynch et al., 2004). Income inequality has a long-term detrimental effect on individual mortality risk (Zheng, 2012). Moreover, welfare states play a more prominent role in the composition of public spending and total economic activity than ever before (Starke et al, 2016). Thus the distribution of public resources must continue to be monitored to alleviate global inequities.

In this regard, social and healthcare services constitute significant aspects of public expenditures. Figure 1.1 highlights the fact that pensions and healthcare spending account for much of the public social spending in OECD countries. Countries on average spend more on cash benefits [12% of gross domestic product (GDP)] than on healthcare and social services (around 8% of GDP). Of public social expenditures, just over 70% in Italy, Poland, and Portugal and 80% in Greece involve cash benefits. In contrast, this proportion was just over 40% in Chile, South Korea, and Mexico and 35% in Iceland. Public pension payments also account for much of social spending. Healthcare receives the second largest amount of spending, behind pensions, in OECD countries (OECD, 2019). Age structure of the populations, number of elder people in the family, economic/financial crisis, and burden of diseases determines public spending trends for pensions and healthcare services (McCullough et al., 2019).

Countries with high levels of social expenditure have significantly better health outcomes (Bardley et al., 2011). Although the interrelationship between social spending and health outcomes are of great interest to researchers, studies of the association between social service and health outcomes within developed countries are limited; for example, in the United States, it is difficult to compare data on social services spending across states (Bradley et al., 2016).

Public management policies, regional differences, and rural–urban dynamics influence public spending on healthcare (Bates and Santerre, 2013). Moreover, such spending is lower in countries with developing economies than in developed nations, and in underdeveloped economies such as

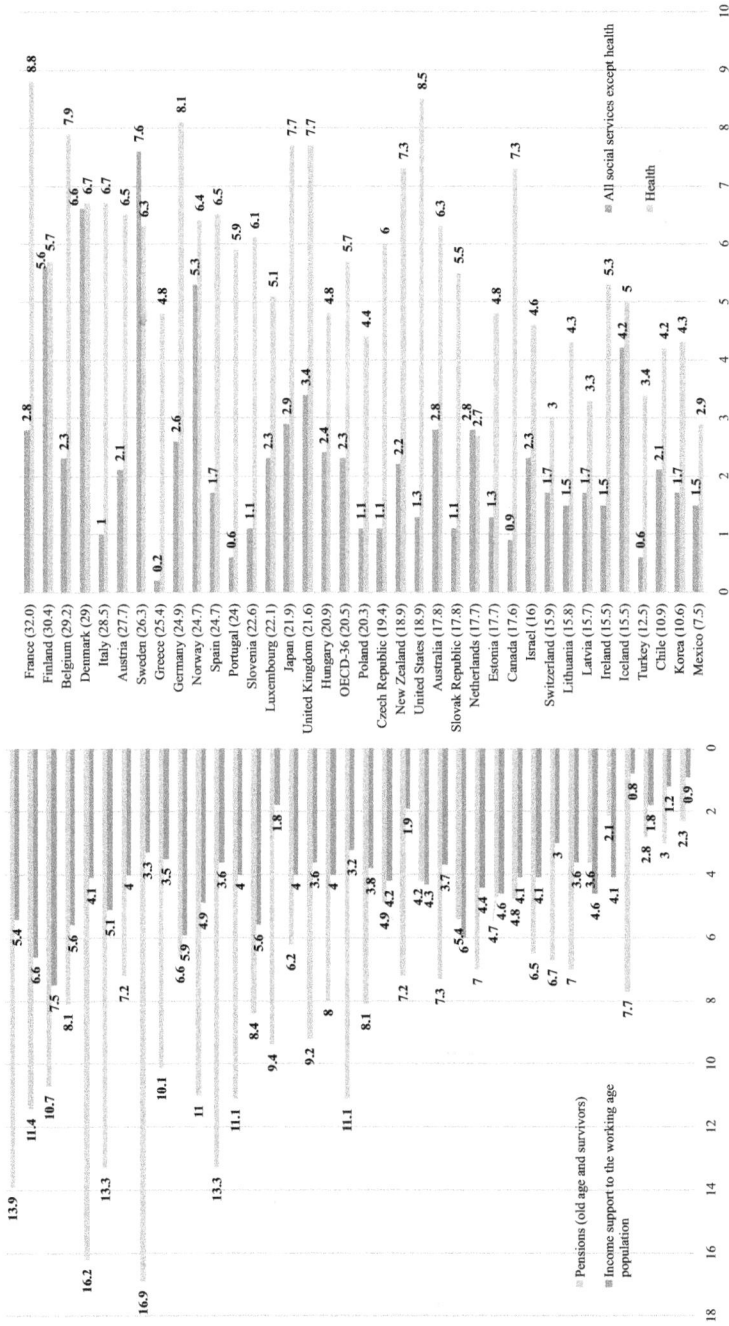

Figure 1.1 Public social expenditure by broad social policy area, in percentage of GDP, 2015/17 or latest year available.

Source: OECD (2019). Public social spending is high in many OECD countries. Social Expenditure Update 2019. Retrieved from: www.oecd.org/social/soc/OECD2019-Social-Expenditure-Update.pdf. Accessed on: 8.11.2019.

African countries, public healthcare expenditures are not handled efficiently (Grigoli and Kapsoli, 2017). In terms of healthcare services and health outcomes, developing countries are worse off than advanced ones. A child is expected to live about 15 years longer in an average advanced economy than in an emerging or developing one. The mortality rate for children younger than 5 years in emerging and developing economies is 11 times the rate in advanced economies (Grigoli and Kapsoli, 2017). Differences in immunization rates are stark; however, humanitarian organizations have helped provide vaccines in underdeveloped nations (Grigoli and Kapsoli, 2017). Public health expenditure for immunization and essential primary health services must be monitored continuously to offset global inequities.

Pharmaceutical expenditures constitute a major part of health expenditures. Drug discovery and development industry is under the pressure to become more efficient and develop better and cheaper drugs at a faster rate (Tyebjee and Hardin, 2004). Today, individualized strategies encompass disease prevention, diagnosis, and treatment strategies. Moreover, data mining and personalized medicine are paving the way to improve the concern for equity (Estabe et al., 2016).

Personalized medicine benefits from the ongoing research on the human body and from genetic knowledge, the idea that health is defined by genetics, and the idea that individual citizens are responsible for their own health status (Savard, 2013). The success of personalized medicine depends on the following: (1) the availability of big data and the role of biomedical informatics in personalized medicine; (2) the involvement of interdisciplinary teams in the development of personalized therapeutic approaches; and (3) electronic medical record systems and clinical data warehouses (Estabe et al., 2016).

In personalized medicine, big data are used to examine health equity from a different point of view. As the complete mapping of the human genome, many genetic variations have been identified. Scientists continue to develop diagnostic tests and treatment modalities that improve an individual patient's response to treatment in accordance with his or her unique genetic profile. Genetic technologies emphasize the need to incorporate genetic information into traditional socioeconomic determinants of health (Estabe et al., 2016). Ethical issues and the incorporation of genetics and genomics into personalized medicine can be considered from equity and accessibility perspectives; there is the risk that these technologies are available only to wealthy populations (Mardis, 2010). Researchers in the field of public health genomics are thus concerned about equity in personalized medicine. It is important to consider the heterogeneity of backgrounds, abilities, and resources of populations with different incomes to modify pricing and develop low-cost personalized medicine programs (Budin-Ljøsne and Harris, 2015).

It is believed that developments in genomic sciences and personalized medicine will alleviate health problems in developing nations; these problems range from tropical diseases to noncommunicable diseases to the effects of globalization on health. Pharmacogenetics and personalized medicine help in diagnosis, prevention, and treatment of infectious and chronic diseases through new interventions, better assessment of responses to drugs, and, ultimately, more efficient healthcare delivery. To improve benefits of personalized medicine for developing countries, it is important to build public trust, adopt multidisciplinary approaches to research, develop ethical and regulatory frameworks, and incorporate all stakeholders – healthcare providers and users – in decision and policy-making processes (Pang, 2009). Additionally, the generation of genotype profiles for population groups helps researchers incorporate pharmacogenetics into national drug formularies. Pharmacogenetics will be useful and essential in the future for the developing world (Roederer and McLeod, 2010). In developing countries, it is important to promote the integration of genetic information into the public health decision-making process, enhance the understanding of pharmacogenetics, and provide guidelines for medication prioritization through the use of pharmacogenetic information (Roederer and McLeod, 2010).

Health system differences and equity in health system

International health systems comparison is of great interest to different actors in health policy (Varabyova and Schreyögg, 2013). Decision-making in healthcare is a complex phenomenon (Cleemput et al., 2008) and every country has different financing and healthcare delivery systems. The inequalities in healthcare exist in many healthcare systems; however, their forms and origins vary. Achieving equal access to healthcare services has been a critical objective for many healthcare systems aiming to close gaps in health outcomes between rich and poor (Tangcharoensathien et al., 2015). The primary goal is included into health system performance frameworks developed by international decision-making authorities such as WHO and the OECD (Sözmen and Ünal, 2016).

Governments, patients, providers, payers, and medical technology firms play critical roles in the development of global healthcare. Additionally, healthcare policymaking is affected by local and global policies and planning activities (Thomas et al., 2015). Although many countries have a public healthcare system, each country has its own healthcare system owing to disagreement in politics, the need for regularity and population needs. Therefore, implementing a uniform healthcare management policy in every country is difficult because of the differences between the countries (Mills, 2014).

Income is one of the primary discriminative factors of any country in terms of differences in health services accessibility and utilization. Moreover, this is the most significant factor that explains the differences in the level and growth of healthcare expenditure across countries (Eikemo et al., 2008).

Therefore, the earlier research focused primarily on measuring the size of the income elasticity of healthcare, and its policy implications for the financing and distribution of healthcare resources (Baltagi and Moscone, 2010).

Developing country experiences show that health inequalities rise according to increase in per capita income of the households (Wagstaff, 2002). Therefore, it can be clearly stated that income is a determining factor in the level of development. People living in more developed countries, such as OECD countries, have comparatively higher incomes and higher socio-economic status. These high-income countries help low- and middle-income countries (LMICs) improve their socioeconomic status and health systems (Niessen et al., 2018). As a result, there is an increasing number of studies focused on the income and living conditions of people in the underdeveloped and developing countries (Gottret and Schieber, 2006).

Besides the income level, the quality of healthcare services is another discriminative factor of global health systems and the reason for equity differences. Populations living in developed countries have an advantage regarding access to new health technologies and drugs (Drummond et al., 2013). Thus, measuring the level of quality, accessibility, and equity in healthcare services must be the primary concern of health policymakers and planners to make health services available for all (Thomas et al., 2015). Nonetheless, measuring the quality of healthcare is a global issue. In this regard, the countries are attempting to improve the performance of healthcare systems through enhanced patient-centered care, use of health technology assessment (HTA), and coordination of care (OECD, 2010).

Measuring the quality and performance of a healthcare system has garnered interest because of rising costs, an aging population, and increased medical errors and inequalities. Healthcare quality and performance measurement have undergone reforms to improve the health sector and make healthcare safer and equal to all (Mattke et al., 2006). WHO and the OECD play a significant role in improving the performance of healthcare systems. These organizations publish books and reports about how to measure, assess, and improve the performance of healthcare systems. Such publications make significant contributions toward the improvement of the equity, quality, and performance of healthcare around the world (Arah et al., 2006).

Comparison of the equity performance of health systems is intriguing given the substantial differences between them regarding the financing and organization of healthcare (Lu et al., 2007). Sustainability is one of the main motivations for health policymakers to ensure equity in the health system. This is generally regarded as a dynamic process of continuous improvement. Furthermore, sustainability is the only way of providing continuous improvement in healthcare (Fleiszer et al., 2015).

Encouraging healthcare innovations and sustainability, especially for new technology areas such as pharmaceuticals and medical devices, should be the priority of healthcare policymakers in LMICs (Holeman et al., 2016).

LMICs have poor financial resources. According to the World Bank's classification of national income, these countries are those with a gross national income (GNI) per capita of between $996 and $3895; upper middle-income economies are those with a GNI per capita of between $3896 and $12,055; and high-income economies are those with a GNI per capita of $12,056 or more (World Bank, 2019). Financial resource constraints have limited innovation in LMICs.

Globalization and increasing inequalities in income, the distribution of health resources and consideration of income inequalities are the main concerns of policymakers (Wade, 2004; Marmot, 2005). Moreover, global recession and unemployment cause a drop in the demand; unemployment and economic distress strain the public budgets and increase the demand for public health services (Mladovsky et al., 2012).

Economic crisis, political instabilities, and rural–urban differences are the main determinants of distributive policies in healthcare. Healthcare system dynamics also affect the redistribution of health resources. The origins of the healthcare system are a determinant of resource distribution in healthcare (Hosseinpoor et al., 2015). Traditionally, the main healthcare policies in this system are the "*Beveridge*" system, based on the National Health System, and the "*Bismarck*" system, based on social insurance and socially inclusive policies. Industrialized countries are faced with similar problems when improving their health system performance. However, significant differences exist between the two systems. The Beveridge-type systems have sought to improve patient choice and reduce inefficiencies in health services usage whereas the Bismarck-type systems focus more on cost control to finance their health reform plans (Or et al., 2010).

On the other hand, healthcare is becoming more complicated owing to breakthroughs in medical science, innovations in medical and drug development technologies, and improvements in clinical practices (Rouse and Serban, 2014). Current systems are no longer adequate for dealing with healthcare problems in this complex environment. Moreover, it is not possible to classify world health nowadays, such as East versus West or North versus South (WHO, 2006).

Apparently, before the 1990s, the assessment of health policies focused on technical content and design factors, but these perspectives neglected the involvement of different healthcare professionals and processes in healthcare decision-making (Li and Benton, 1996). In the early 1990s, several analysts called for a new approach for health policy analysis in LMICs. This new approach requires collaborative policymaking for global healthcare systems (Gilson and Raphaely, 2008).

Over the last several decades, debates on global health have garnered the attention of healthcare policymakers. Global healthcare promotes broader thinking regarding healthcare systems and ways to transfer knowledge internationally (Wensing and Grol, 2019). Health trends and technologies are shaping current health policies, decision-making, and equity, which would lead to different institutions and organizations sharing physical, financial, and human healthcare resources (Mills, 2014).

Health trends and equity

Healthcare is one of the fastest growing areas of the world economy (Emami and Doolen, 2015). The rapidly growing complexity and technology in healthcare enable an increase in the level of general health expenditure and demand for access to modern technologies. These developments have incentivized the interest of health professionals regarding HTA in LMICs (Dankó, 2014). HTA includes pharmaceuticals, medical devices, clinical procedures, surgical interventions, and diagnostics. Pharmaceuticals and medical devices are the two main areas of focus in HTA studies in most countries (Dankó and Petrova, 2014).

Despite an increased interest in technology management in healthcare, it is difficult to implement and develop a process for HTA in LMICs conclusively (Bijlmakers et al., 2017). In other words, there is a scarcity of knowledge about professional HTA in LMICs. A balanced perspective is an advisable strategy to improve the degree of professionality of HTA studies globally.

Balanced scorecard (BSC) is a strategic management tool for multidimensional management of health technologies. Specifically, in their HTA studies, LMICs need to follow their own approaches in the adaptation of BSC models (Dankó, 2014).

BSC enables to assess health technology management performance not only from a financial but also from a nonfinancial perspective (Kaplan and Norton, 1996). To clarify, during the adaptation process of BSC model to HTA, the critical question according to the financial perspective is: "To succeed in an HTA study, how much money should we pay this new health technology?" Patient satisfaction is one of the subjective performance measures of health systems. Thus, including patient satisfaction into HTA studies is necessary to answer patient needs related to health technology trends. Additionally, this is one of the ways of understanding the reasons behind increasing health expenditures (Fenton et al., 2012).

According to the customer perspective, the crucial question is: "To achieve our vision and strategies in the HTA market, how should we appear to patients and other stakeholders?" The most critical question of health technologies, which enable to incorporate equity into the HTA process is: "To satisfy our stakeholders and customers, what business processes should we excel at?" This question is related to the internal business perspective of the BSC model. The motivation behind health reforms is to ensure equity, which is the only way to understand health consumers better.

Finally, according to the learning and growth perspective, the critical question is "To achieve our vision, how will we sustain our ability to change and improve HTA" (Atkinson, 2006). Effective management of health trends is possible only with institutionalized and integrated approaches. Therefore, it is advisable for LMICs to have a broader perspective and consider not only the financial perspective but also the nonfinancial perspective when managing health technologies and trends. It can be clearly stated that a balanced management perspective will help to solve health system problems and follow health trends in the longer run (Aidemark, 2002). Additionally, this perspective enables seeing the big picture and effectively forms a detailed conceptual framework for managing technology and other healthcare resources. Adopting a broader perspective by not only considering financial indicators but also the nonfinancial indicators will enable to make better plans to control the increase in health expenditures (Omran et al., 2019).

The balanced perspective provides significant benefits when equity is considered the primary concern for a better design of the health system. This perspective is also an innovative and broader way of policymaking and cost control in healthcare. Figure 1.2 gives a brief overview of the adaptation of BSC to HTA. Dimensions of BSC is adapted from Drummond et al. (2012), Dankó (2014), Zelman et al. (2003), and Gurd and Gao (2008).

Perspectives and measures of BSC provide potential benefits regarding the effective management of health technologies in LMICs. Policymakers in LMICs need to consider costs, income and amount of research income, and profits of new technologies for effective management in healthcare dynamics (Jakovljevic and Getzen, 2016).

Internal business perspective includes cost-effectiveness and budget impact analysis, which are fundamental analysis tools of new HTA. Customer and stakeholder analysis is another dimension of effective management of health technologies and trends. Understanding customer needs and necessities is critical for better health technology management (Drummond et al., 2013). Incorporating principles of equity into the customer perspective will enhance customer satisfaction and answer their needs better.

Learning and growth is another perspective of BSC, which includes staff education and training health programs about epidemiology and biostatistics. Learning, growth, and new drug research have shaped the evolution of the industrial and market structure of the pharmaceutical sector (Grant et al., 2019). More focus on learning, growth and continuous monitoring and sharing of new drug information are essential strategies for improving the efficiency of the pharmaceutical market, which is one of the most costly areas in the healthcare industry (Paul et al., 2010). In the pharmaceutical market, equity should be one of the primary concerns. The distributional analysis of pharmaceutical expenditures is of great interest to healthcare policymakers. Managers in the pharmaceutical industry should be aware of quality and cost-effectiveness in the production, which constitute the dimensions of internal business and financial management of BSC (García-Valderrama et al., 2009).

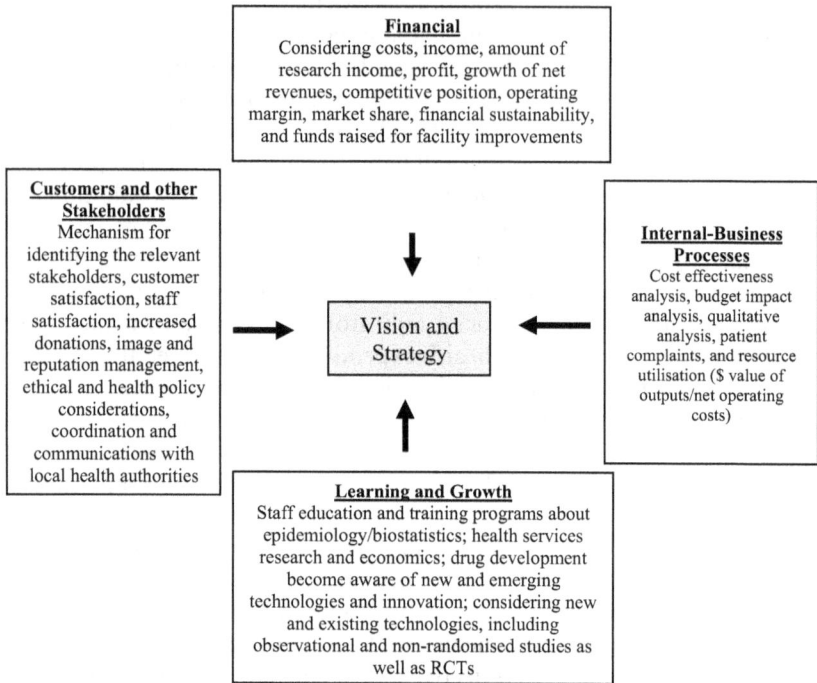

Financial
Considering costs, income, amount of
research income, profit, growth of net
revenues, competitive position, operating
margin, market share, financial sustainability,
and funds raised for facility improvements

**Customers and other
Stakeholders**
Mechanism for
identifying the relevant
stakeholders, customer
satisfaction, staff
satisfaction, increased
donations, image and
reputation management,
ethical and health policy
considerations,
coordination and
communications with
local health authorities

Vision and
Strategy

**Internal-Business
Processes**
Cost effectiveness
analysis, budget impact
analysis, qualitative
analysis, patient
complaints, and resource
utilisation ($ value of
outputs/net operating
costs)

Learning and Growth
Staff education and training programs about
epidemiology/biostatistics; health services
research and economics; drug development
become aware of new and emerging
technologies and innovation; considering new
and existing technologies, including
observational and non-randomised studies as
well as RCTs

Figure 1.2 Adaptation of BSC to HTA (perspectives and measures) for LMICs.

Sources: Adapted from Drummond et al. (2012), Danko (2014), Zelman et al. (2003), Gurd and Gao (2008).

Developed economies have made advancements in drug development and research technologies. However, developing and underdeveloped countries require more knowledge and policy support to develop their potential in the pharmaceutical market. Additionally, the pharmaceutical market is one of the most competitive markets in the world (Lei et al., 2016). Thus, developed countries should provide more support to the developing countries so that these nations can enhance financial management, improve research and development of BSCs, and develop pharmaceutical strategies (Elovainio, 2010).

Therefore, effective market regulations are essential for the sustainability of this market and enabling accessibility of new drugs for the vulnerable population. Obviously, considering equity is a significant concern for health policymakers who are regulating the pharmaceutical market (Feyzrakhmanova and Gurdgiev, 2016). Rational usage of resources and effective resource planning is an integral part of this process. Thus, specific HTA analysis techniques such as cost-effectiveness analysis should be an integral part of the assessment of the new technologies in the pharmaceutical market (Leung et al., 2013). On the other hand, however, health professionals are faced with struggles during the adaptation process of new health technologies and innovations (Jha and Topol, 2016). Therefore, it is highly advisable that health policymakers from LMICs prepare specific education programs and continually monitor the level of usage of advanced health technologies to enable easy adaptation of innovations in healthcare.

Equity is the main principle to ensure a sustainable healthcare system. Socially inclusive policies and insurance coverage enhancement in society will provide significant benefits for the vulnerable groups. Thus, social inclusiveness and equity must be the primary concern of health policymakers in LMICs because inclusive policies will enhance access to pharmaceuticals. The following section emphasizes the importance of social inclusiveness and equity in healthcare.

Social inclusiveness and equity in healthcare

Most health reforms and innovations in healthcare are aiming to reform the access, utilization and distribution of health benefits to the population (Kutzin and Sparkes, 2016). The primary motivation of these reforms is to ensure financial protection of the population at a disadvantage. Achieving a socially inclusive health system incentivizes health policymakers in developing countries to use healthcare resources better (Atun et al., 2016).

The motivation behind socially inclusive policies is to ensure equity in the distribution of healthcare resources considering the income and other socioeconomic differences of the population (Thomson et al., 2018). Strengthening primary health services, increasing health insurance coverage, and considering health benefits in vulnerable groups are the major strategies that can provide equity in healthcare (Bloom, 2001).

However, the concern regarding health system equity is not the same in every country. The main concerns and health system differences of the European countries and the US are determining factors. New technological developments and advanced research form part of the health technology market in the US, whereas the European market is based on the social insurance system (Drummond et al., 2005; Drummond et al., 1992). Thus, improving the quality and accessibility of primary care is the main objective of the health system of European countries. The two-sided nature of health system dynamics brings on to the table significant differences between the US and Europe regarding competitive market regulations, such as pharmaceuticals and medical devices. There is a strong notion of equity among European countries. However, the high costs of technology and research and development show that equity has become less important for the healthcare system in the US. The US is the leader among developed countries regarding increasing healthcare costs. Moreover, it is the leader in innovation-based economies and a pioneering country in research and development of new health technologies (Banta, 2003). High costs and prices affect the health consumers, thereby leading to inevitable inequalities regarding access, utilization, and expenditure of health services (Torbica et al., 2018). Despite the surges in costs highlighting the importance of effective management of health resources, the relationship between equity and effectiveness is controversial (Karsu and Morton, 2015). Striving for equity does not necessarily result in high healthcare costs. In every country, policymakers need to be aware of the burden of health expenditures and attempt to provide equal distribution of welfare (WHO, 2013b).

In other words, because of the differences in healthcare system dynamics, private sector and competition are the primary concerns of the US health system, which has led to the development of a competitive health technology market in the US. Consequently, high expenses in healthcare bring high costs and threaten the financial sustainability of the US health system (Papanicolas et al., 2018).

Although the US is undoubtedly a leader in the competitive health technology market regarding the development of recent health technologies and the diagnosis and treatment of life-threatening diseases, the increased health expenditure moves away from the principle of equity in healthcare (OECD, 2019). Therefore, the vulnerable groups in the population have been placed at a disadvantage owing to this and healthcare system reforms have become one of the primary agendas of health policymakers. By contrast, countries belonging to the Bismark system, such as the UK, provide little choice for health consumers, and their core principle is social equity (Torbica et al., 2018).

Therefore, healthcare system dynamics differ among developed countries and the level of their concern regarding equity is markedly different. On the other hand, developing countries have adopted different healthcare system dynamics for the effective use of limited health resources. Therefore, the primary motivation of health policymakers in most developing countries is the measurement and continuous monitoring of the level of equity in healthcare (Forster et al., 2019). Furthermore, rural and urban differences in health are more marked in developing countries. Over the years, the debate on the equitable allocation of financial resources in healthcare has focused on the allocation from a national to a regional level. Therefore, an examination of inequalities by considering regional differences is essential to ensure a more sustainable healthcare system globally (Asante et al., 2006).

Nonetheless, a strong primary healthcare system is one of the ways of efficiently managing the health resources and creating a more responsive health system. However, empirical studies regarding equity in primary healthcare systems are limited (Hone et al., 2017).

There is scant evidence against which to evaluate the equity performance of the health systems of the high-income economies in Asia (Lu et al., 2007). Cross-country comparisons suggest that broader health coverage and pooled financing helped to expand access to necessary care with improvements in population health, especially for poor people (Moreno-Serra and Smith, 2012). Specific areas of health services, such as maternal care, need more attention in terms of equity. Knowledge about equity in the utilization of maternal healthcare in developing countries is lacking. Moreover, income and wealth status are the crucial factors that determine who receives care. Race, ethnicity, and religion have had statistically significant effects on the use of maternal care in developing countries (Caliskan et al., 2015). A study on equity of utilization of in- and outpatient services in Turkey revealed inequities in the use of healthcare services in 2010, 2012, and 2014. Policy advice is needed to improve insurance coverage of poor citizens and to protect disadvantaged segments of the population (Başar et al., 2018). In this regard, unification of health financing systems and ensuring universal health coverage is one of the common strategies to curtail healthcare inequities in developing countries. Several middle-income countries, such as Turkey, Brazil, Mexico, and Thailand, have sought to unify health insurance systems with universal health coverage along with LMICs, including China, Indonesia, Philippines, and South Africa (Tirgil et al., 2018). Early experience with universal health coverage in Turkey have shown that non-contributory health insurance programs, such as the Green Card scheme, increase poor people's access to healthcare services. Turkey's experience provides important lessons for countries whose aim is to develop inclusive health coverage to protect vulnerable groups (Tirgil et al., 2018).

With improvement in the distribution of healthcare and better financial protection, the level of satisfaction from health services will increase (Lu and Hsiao, 2003). Strong primary care is one of the main indicators of success of universal healthcare. According to recent study findings from Turkey, strengthening of primary care with the Family Medicine Model improved the level of patient satisfaction with care (Sparkes et al., 2019). In this regard, it is highly advisable for health policymakers in developing countries to build a strong primary care system to improve the level of patient satisfaction with care and to improve quality of care (Andaleeb, 2001). Moreover, it is highly advisable that health policymakers incorporate national, consistent user satisfaction surveys of the health systems into the performance assessment processes to respond better to the health consumer's necessities (Kersnik, 2001).

In this regard, national user satisfaction surveys are the starting point to get subjective performance assessment of health services. To conclude, social inclusiveness and equity are the primary agendas of every health reform experience. However, to make the equity dream come true, strong political support and awareness of the potential benefits of an inclusive and responsive health system are critical (Elovainio, 2010). Although equity is one of the most significant challenges of public health, there is a lack of knowledge about the methodology of equity and examination of pharmaceutical expenses, which are the high-cost areas in healthcare services, especially in LMICs (Oortwijn et al., 2010).

This book will now examine equity in the distribution of pharmaceutical expenditures under the health reform experience by focusing on one of the LMICs, which is Turkey. The chapters that follow explain in detail international comparisons of equity in healthcare services (Chapter 2), equity in health services and specific policy advice for developing countries (Chapter 3), equity lessons learned from pharmerging countries (Chapter 4), equity in health services in emerging markets similar to Turkey (Chapter 5), health reform in Turkey and inclusive policies (Chapter 6), measurement of the level of equity in healthcare services (Chapter 7), equity in pharmaceutical expenditures under health reform in Turkey (Chapter 8), advice for health policymakers to consider equity in the distribution of pharmaceutical expenditures and pharmaceutical market design (Chapter 9).

References

Acemoglu D, Ucer M. (2015) The ups and downs of Turkish growth, 2002–2015: Political dynamics, the European Union and the institutional slide. The National Bureau of Economic Research. NBER Working Paper. No. 21608.

Agartan TI. (2015) Explaining large-scale policy change in the Turkish Health Care System: Ideas, institutions, and political actors. *Journal of Health Politics, Policy and Law* 40(5):971–999.

Aidemark LG. (2002) The meaning of balanced scorecards in the health care organisation. *Financial Accountability & Management* 17(1):23–40.

Akdağ R. (2003) Health Transformation Programme. Ministry of Health, Ankara, Turkey.

Anand S. (2002) The concern for equity in health. *Journal of Epidemiology & Community Health* 56(7):485–487.

Andaleeb SS. (2001) Service quality perceptions and patient satisfaction: A study of hospitals in a developing country. *Social Science & Medicine* 52(9):1359–1370.

Arah OA, Westert GP, Hurst J, Klazinga N.S. (2006) A conceptual framework for the OECD health care quality indicators project. *International Journal for Quality in Health Care* 18(1):5–13.

Asante AD, Zwi AB, Ho MT. (2006) Equity in resource allocation for health: A comparative study of the Ashanti and Northern Regions of Ghana. *Health Policy* 78(2–3):135–148.

Atkinson H. (2006) Strategy implementation: A role for the balanced scorecard? *Management Decision* 44(10):1441–1460.

Atun R, Aydın S, Chakraborty S, Sümer S, Aran M, Gürol I, Nazlıoğlu S, Özgülcü S, Aydoğan U, Ayar B, Dilmen U, Akdağ R. (2013) Universal health coverage in Turkey: Enhancement of equity. *The Lancet* 382(9886):65–99.

Atun R, Chaumont C, Fitchett JR, Haakenstad A, Kaberuka D. (2016) Poverty alleviation and the economic benefits of investing in health. Harvard T.H. Chan School of Public Health. Forum for Finance Ministers, 2006. April 11 2016.

Baltagi BH, Moscone F. (2010) Health care expenditure and income in the OECD reconsidered: Evidence from panel data. *Economic Modelling* 27(4):804–811.

Bambas Nolen L, Braveman P, Dachs JNW, Delgado I, Gakidou E, Moser K, Rolfe L, Vega J, Zarowsky C. (2005) Strengthening health information systems to address health equity challenges. *Bulletin of the World Health Organization* 83(8):597–603.

Banta D. (2003) The development of health technology assessment. *Health Policy* 63(2):121–132.

Başar D, Öztürk S, Çakmak İ. (2018) An application of the behavioral model to the utilization of health care services in Turkey: A focus on equity. *PharmacoEconomics* doi: 10.2298/PAN171121006B.

Bates LJ, Santerre RE. (2013) Does regionalization of local public health services influence public spending levels and allocative efficiency? *Regional Science and Urban Economics* 43(2):209–219.

Baum F, Fisher M. (2010) Health equity and sustainability: Extending the work of the Commission on the Social Determinants of Health. *Critical Public Health* 20(3):311–322.

Beauchamp TL, Childress JF (eds) (1994) *Principles of biomedical ethics*. Oxford University Press: New York, pp. 326–359.

Bijlmakers L, Mueller D, Kahveci R, Chen Y, van der Wilt G. (2017) Integrate-HTA: A low- and middle-income country perspective. *International Journal of Technology Assessment in Health Care* 33(5):599–604.

Bloom G. (2001) Equity in health in unequal societies: Meeting health needs in contexts of social change. *Health Policy* 57:205–224.

Bradley EH, Elkins BR, Herrin J, Elbel B. (2011) Health and social services expenditures: Associations with health outcomes. *BMJ Quality & Safety* 20(10):826–831.

Bradley EH. Canavan M, Rogan E, Talbert-Slagle K, Ndumele C, Taylor L, Curry LA. (2016) Variation in health outcomes: The role of spending on social services, public health and health care, 2000–09. *Health Affairs* (Millwood) 35(5):760–768.

Braveman P, Gruskin S. (2003) Defining equity in health. *Journal of Epidemiology & Community Health* 57(4):254–258.

Brown S, Hole AR, Kilic D. (2014) Out-of-pocket health care expenditure in Turkey: Analysis of the 2003–2008 Household Budget Surveys. *Economic Modelling* 41:211–218.

Budin-Ljøsne I, Harris JR. (2015) Ask not what personalized medicine can do for you – Ask what you can do for personalized medicine. *Public Health Genomics* 18(3):131–138.

Caliskan Z, Kılıç D, Öztürk S, Atılgan E. (2015) Equity in maternal health care service utilization: A systematic review for developing countries. *International Journal of Public Health* 60(7):815–825.

Cash-Gibson L, Rojas-Gualdrón DF, Pericàs JM, Benach J. (2018) Inequalities in global health inequalities research: A 50-year bibliometric analysis (1966–2015). *PLoS ONE* 13(1):e0191901.

Cleemput I, Neyt M, Thiry N, De Leat CD, Leys M. (2008) Threshold values for cost-effectiveness in health care. The Belgian Health Care Knowledge Center, KCE Reports 100. 2008. Belgium.

Commission on Social Determinants of Health (CSDH) (2008) Closing the gap in a generation: Health equity through action on the social determinants of health: Final report of the Commission on Social Determinants of Health. World Health Organization: Geneva, Switzerland.

Dankó D, Petrova G. (2014) Health technology assessment in the Balkans: Opportunities for a balanced drug assessment system. *Biotechnology & Biotechnological Equipment* 28 (6):1181–1189.

Dankó D. (2014) Health technology assessment in middle-income countries: Recommendations for a balanced assessment system. *Journal of Market Access & Health Policy* 2:1–10.

Deaton A. (2003) Health, inequality, and economic development. *Journal of Economic Literature* 41(1):113–158.

Doyle SK, Chang AM, Levy P, Rising KL. (2019) Achieving health equity in hypertension management through addressing the social determinants of health. *Current Hypertension Reports* 21(58):1–6.

Drummond M, Bloom BS, Carrin G, Hillman AL, Hutchings HC, Knill-jones R, De Pouvourville G, Torfs K. (1992) Issues in the cross-national assessment of health technology. *International Journal of Technology Assessment in Health Care* 8(4):670–682.

Drummond M, Manca A, Sculpher M. (2005) Increasing the generalizability of economic evaluations: Recommendations for the design, analysis, and reporting of studies. *International Journal of Technology Assessment in Health Care* 21(2):165–171.

Drummond M, Neumann P, Jönsson B, Luce B, Schwartz JS, Siebert U, Sullivan SD. (2012) Can we reliably benchmark health technology assessment organizations? *International Journal of Health Technology Assessment* 28(2):159–165.

Drummond M, Tarricone R, Torbica A. (2013) Assessing the added value of health technologies: Reconciling different perspectives. *Value in Health* 16(1):S7-S13.

Eikemo TA, Bambra C, Judge K, Ringdal K. (2008) Welfare state regimes and differences in self-perceived health in Europe: A multilevel analysis. *Social Science & Medicine* 66(11):2281–2295.

Elovainio R. (2010) Performance incentives for health in high-income countries key issues and lessons learned. World Health Report. Background Paper. 32. www.who.int/healthsystems/topics/financing/healthreport/32PBF.pdf?ua=1. Accessed on: 24.2.2019.

Emami S, Doolen TL. (2015) Healthcare performance measurement: Identification of metrics for the learning and growth balanced scorecard perspective. *International Journal of Industrial Engineering* 22(4):426–437.

Estape ES, Mays MH, Sternke EA. (2016) Translation in data mining to advance personalized medicine for health equity. *Intelligent Information Management* 8(1):9–16.

Evans DB, Hsu J, Boerma T. (2013) Universal health coverage and universal access. *Bulletin of the World Health Organization* 91(8):546–546A.

Evans T, Whitehead M, Diderichsen F, Bhuiya A, Wirth M. eds. (2001) *Challenging inequities in health: From ethics to action.* New York: Oxford University Press, UK.

Fenton JJ, Jerant AF, Bertakis KD, Franks P. (2012) The cost of satisfaction a national study of patient satisfaction, health care utilization, expenditures, and mortality. *Archives of Internal Medicine* 172(5):405–411.

Feyzrakhmanova M, Gurdgiev C. (2016) Patents and R&D expenditure effects on equity returns in pharmaceutical industry. *Applied Economics Letters* 23(4):278–283.

Fiscella K, Franks P, Gold MR, Clancy CM. (2000) Inequality in quality: Addressing socioeconomic, racial, and ethnic disparities in health care. *JAMA* 283(19):2579–2584.

Fleiszer AR, Semenic SE, Ritchie JA, Richer MC, Denis JL. (2015) The sustainability of healthcare innovations: A concept analysis. *Journal of Advanced Nursing* 71(7):1484–1498.

Forster T, Kentikelenis AE, Stubbs TH, King LP. (2019) Globalization and health equity: The impact of structural adjustment programs on developing countries. *Social Science & Medicine*. https://doi.org/10.1016/j.socscimed.2019.112496.

García-Valderrama T, Mulero-Mendigorri E, Revuelta-Bordoy D. (2009) Relating the perspectives of the balanced scorecard for R&D by means of DEA. *European Journal of Operations Research* 196(3):1177–1189.

Gemmill MC, Thomson S, Mossialos E. (2008) What impact do prescription drug charges have on efficiency and equity? Evidence from high-income countries. *International Journal for Equity in Health Care* 7(12):1–22.

Gilson L, Raphaely N. (2008) The terrain of health policy analysis in low and middle income countries: A review of published literature 1994–2007. *Health Policy and Planning* 23(5):294–307.

Gottret P, Schieber G. (2006) Health financing revisited: A practitioner's guide. The World Bank. https://openknowledge.worldbank.org/handle/10986/7094 License: CC BY 3.0 IGO.

Graham H. (2004) Social determinants and their unequal distribution: Clarifying policy understandings. *Milbank Quarterly* 82(1):101–124.

Grant K, Matousek R, Meyer M, Tzeremes NG. (2019) Research and development spending and technical efficiency: Evidence from biotechnology and pharmaceutical sector. *International Journal of Production Research* doi:10.1080/00207543.2019.1671623.

Grigoli F, Kapsoli J. (2017) Waste not, want not: The efficiency of health expenditure in emerging and developing economies. *Review of Development Economics* 22(1):384–403.

Gurd B, Gao T. (2008) Lives in the balance: An analysis of the balanced scorecard (BSC) in healthcare organizations. *International Journal of Productivity and Performance Management* 57(1):6–21.

Hall RL, Jacobson PD. (2018) Examining whether the health-in-all-policies approach promotes health equity. *Health Affairs* (Millwood) 37(3):364–370.

Holeman I, Patricia Cookson T, Pagliari C. (2016) Digital technology for health sector governance in low and middle income countries: A scoping review. *Journal of Global Health* 6(2):1–11.

Hone T, Gurol-Urgancı I, Millett C, Başara B, Akdağ R, Atun R. (2017) Effect of primary health care reforms in Turkey on health service utilization and user satisfaction. *Health Policy and Planning* 32(1):57–67.

Hosseinpoor AR, Bergen N, Schlotheuber A. (2015) Promoting health equity: WHO health inequality monitoring at global and national levels. *Global Health Action* 8(29034):1–8.

Jakovljevic M, Getzen TE. (2016) Growth of global health spending share in low and middle income countries. *Frontiers in Pharmacology* 7:1–4.

Jha S, Topol EJ. (2016) Adapting to artificial intelligence radiologists and pathologists as information specialists. *JAMA* 316(22):2353–2354.

Kaplan RS, Norton DP. (1996) Linking the balanced scorecard to strategy. *California Management Review* 39(1):53–79.

Karsu Ö, Morton A. (2015) Inequity averse optimization in operational research. *European Journal of Operational Research* 245(2):343–359.

Kersnik J. (2001) Determinants of customer satisfaction with the health care system, with the possibility to choose a personal physician and with a family doctor in a transition country. *Health Policy* 57(2):155–164.

Khaled MA, Makdissi P, Yazbeck M. (2018) Income-related health transfers principles and orderings of joint distributions of income and health. *Journal of Health Economics* 57:315–331.

Kutzin J, Sparkes SP. (2016) [Editorial] Health systems strengthening, universal health coverage, health security and resilience. *Bulletin of the World Health Organization* 94(2):2.

Leach-Kemon K, Chou DP, Schneider MT, Tardif A, Dieleman JL, Brooks BP, Hanlon M, Murray CJ. (2012) The global financial crisis has led to a slowdown in growth of funding to improve health in many developing countries. *Health Affairs* (Millwood) 31(1):228–235.

Lei J. Lin B. Sha S. (2016) Catching-up pattern among countries in science-based industries: A case study in pharmaceutical industry. *Journal of Industrial Integration and Management* 1(1). https://doi.org/10.1142/S2424862216500044. Accessed on: 7.9.2019.

Leung HW, Chan ALF, Leung MS, Lu CL. (2013) Systematic review and quality assessment of cost-effectiveness analysis of pharmaceutical therapies for advanced colorectal cancer. *Annals of Pharmacotherapy* 47(4):506–518.

Levey SM, Miller BF, deGruy FV. (2012) Behavioral health integration: An essential element of population-based healthcare redesign. *Translational Behavioral Medicine* 2(3):364–371.

Li LX, Benton WC. (1996) Performance measurement criteria in health care organizations: Review and future research directions. *European Journal of Operational Research* 93(3):449–468.

Liaropoulos L, Goranitis I. (2015) Health care financing and the sustainability of health systems. *International Journal for Equity in Health* 14(80):1–4.

Liu GG, Zhao Z, Cai R, Yamada T, Yamada T. (2002) Equity in health care access to: Assessing the urban health insurance reform in China. *Social Science & Medicine* 55(10):1779–1794.

Lu JFR, Hsiao WC. (2003) Does universal health insurance make health care unaffordable? Lessons from Taiwan. *Health Affairs* (Millwood) 22(3):77–88.

Lu JR, Leung GM, Kwon S, Tin KYK, van Doorslaer E, O'Donnell O. (2007) Horizontal equity in health care utilization evidence from three high-income Asian economies. *Social Science & Medicine* 64(1):199–212.

Lynch J, Smith GD, Harper S, Hillemeier M, Ross N, Kaplan GA, Wolfson M. (2004) Is income inequality a determinant of population health? Part 1. A systematic review. *Milbank Quarterly* 82(1):5–99.

Mardis ER. (2010) The $1000 genome, the $100,000 analysis? *Genome Medicine* 2(84):1–3.

Marmot M. (2005) Social determinants of health inequalities. *The Lancet* 365(9464):1099–1104.

Mattke S, Epstein AM, Leatherman S. (2006) The OECD health care quality indicators project: History and background. *International Journal for Quality in Health Care* 18(1):1–4

McCullough JM, Singh SR, Leider JP. (2019) The importance of governmental and nongovernmental investments in public health and social services for improving community health outcomes. *Journal of Public Health Management and Practice* 25(4):348–356.

Meng, Q., Fang, H., Liu, X., Yuan, B., Xu, J. (2015) Consolidating the social health insurance schemes in China: Towards an equitable and efficient health system. *The Lancet* 386 (10002):1484–1492.

Mills A. (2014) Health care systems in low- and middle- income countries. *The New England Journal of Medicine* 370(6):552–557.

Ministry of Health (MoH) (2015) Health Statistics Year Book-2015. https://dosyasb. saglik.gov.tr/Eklenti/6118,healthstatisticsyearbook2015pdf.pdf?0. Accessed on: 3.4.2019.

Mladovsky P, Srivastava D, Cylus J, Karanikolos M, Evetovits T, Thomson S, McKee M. (2012) Health policy responses to the financial crisis in Europe. Copenhagen: WHO Regional Office for Europe and European Observatory on Health Systems and Policies.

Moreno-Serra R, Smith PC. (2012) Does progress towards universal health coverage improve population health? *The Lancet* 380(9845):917–923.

Moss J. (2007) Against fairness: Egalitarianism and responsibility. *The Journal of Value Inquiry* 41:309–324.

Niessen LW, Mohan D, Akuoku JK, Mirelman AJ, Ahmed S, Koehlmoss TP. et al. (2018) Tackling socioeconomic inequalities and non-communicable diseases in low-income and middle-income countries under the Sustainable Development agenda. *The Lancet* 391(10134):2036–2046.

O'Donnell O, van Doorslaer E, Wagstaff A, Lindelow M. (2008) Analyzing health equity using household survey data: A guide to techniques and their implementation. World Bank Institute. The World Bank. Washington, D.C.

Omran M, Khallaf A, Gleason K, Tahat Y. (2019) Non-financial performance measures disclosure, quality strategy, and organizational financial performance: A mediating model. Total Quality Management & Business Excellence. doi:10.1080/14783363.2019.1625708.

Onis Z. (2015) Monopolising the centre: The AKP and the uncertain path of Turkish democracy. *The International Spectator* 50(2):22–41.

Oortwijn W, Mathijssen J, Banta D. (2010) The role of health technology assessment on pharmaceutical reimbursement in selected middle-income countries. *Health Policy* 95 (2–3): 174–184.

Or Z, Cases C, Lisac M, Vrangbæk K, Winblad U, Bevan G. (2010) Are health problems systemic? Politics of access and choice under Beveridge and Bismarck systems. *Health Economics Policy and Law* 5(03):269–293.

Organization for Economic Co-operation and Development (OECD). (2017) *New health technologies: Managing access, value and sustainability*. OECD Publishing, Paris. http://dx.doi.org/10.1787/9789264266438-en. Accessed on: 25.2.2019.

Organization for Economic Co-operation and Development (OECD). (2010) OECD health ministerial meeting forum on quality of care, Forum on Quality of Care, Paris 7–8 October 2010 (30 March 2016 date last accessed).

Organization for Economic Co-operation and Development (OECD). (2019) Public social spending is high in many OECD countries. Social Expenditure Update 2019. www.oecd.org/social/soc/OECD2019-Social-Expenditure-Update.pdf. Accessed on: 28.9.2019.

Ottersen OP, Dasgupta J, Blouin C, Buss P, Chongsuvivatwong V, et al. (2014) The political origins of health inequity: Prospects for change. *The Lancet* 383(9917):630–667.

Ozgen-Narci H, Şahin İ, Yıldırım HH. (2015) Financial catastrophe and poverty impacts of out-of-pocket health payments in Turkey. *European Journal of Health Economics* 16 (3):255–270.

Pang T. (2009) Pharmacogenomics and personalized medicine for the developing world – too soon or just-in-time? A personal view from the World Health Organization. *Current Pharmacogenomics and Personalized Medicine* 7(3): 149–157.

Papanicolas I, Woskie LR, Jha AK. (2018) Health care spending in the United States and other high-income countries. *Journal of American Medical Association* 319(10):1024–1039.

Paul SM, Mytelka DS, Dunwiddie CT, Persinger CC, Munos BH, Lindborg SR, Schacht AL. (2010) How to improve R&D productivity: The pharmaceutical industry's grand challenge. *Nature Reviews Drug Discovery* 9:203–214.

Pickett KE, Wilkinson RG. (2015) Income inequality and health: A causal review. *Social Science & Medicine* 128:316–326.

Piroozi B, Rashidian A, Moradi G, Takian A, Ghasri H, Ghadimi T. (2017) Out-of-pocket and informal payment before and after the health transformation plan in Iran: Evidence from hospitals located in Kurdistan, Iran. *International Journal of Health Policy and Management* 6(10):573–586.

Purnell TS, Calhoun EA, Golden SH, Halladay JR, Krok-Schoen JL, Appelhans BM, Cooper LA. (2016) Achieving health equity: Closing the gaps in health care disparities, interventions and research. *Health Affairs* (Millwood) 35(8):1410–1415.

Roederer MW, McLeod HL. (2010) Applying the genome to national drug formulary policy in the developing world. *Pharmacogenomics* 11(5):633–636.

Rouse WB, Serban N. (2014) Understanding and managing the complexity in healthcare (Engineering Systems). MIT Press: USA.

Savard J. (2013) Personalised medicine: A critique on the future of health care. *Journal of Bioethical Inquiry* 10(2):197–203.

Smith MJ, Weinstock D. (2019) Reducing health inequities through intersectoral action: Balancing equity in health with equity for other social goods. *International Journal of Health Policy and Management* 8(1):1–3.

Social Determinants of Health (SDH). (2008) WHO called to return to the declaration of Alma-Ata. World Health Organization. www.who.int/social_determinants/ tools/multimedia/alma_ata/en/ Accessed on: 9.6.2019.

Sözmen K, Ünal B. (2016) Explaining inequalities in health care utilization among Turkish adults: Findings from Health Survey 2008. *Health Policy* 120(1):100–110.

Sparkes SP, Atun R, Bärnighausen T. (2019) The impact of the Family Medicine Model on patient satisfaction in Turkey: Panel analysis with province fixed effects. *PLoS ONE* 14(1):e0210563. https://doi.org/10.1371/journal.

Starke P, Wulfgramm M, Obinger H. (2016) Welfare state transformation across OECD countries: Supply side orientation, individualized outcome risks and dualization. In: Wulfgramm M., Bieber T., Leibfried S. (eds), *Welfare State Transformations and Inequality in OECD Countries*. Transformations of the State. Palgrave Macmillan, London.

Sustainable development knowledge platform: Open working group proposal for sustainable development goals (SDGs). (2014) United Nations Department of Economic and Social Affairs. https://sustainabledevelopment.un.org/sdgsproposal. Accessed on: 9.8.2019.

Tangcharoensathien V, Mills A, Palu T. (2015) Accelerating health equity: The key role of universal health coverage in the Sustainable Development Goals. *BMC Medicine* 13(101):1–5.

Terrelonge SC. (2014) For health, strength, and daily food: The dual impact of remittances and public health expenditure on household health spending and child health outcomes. *The Journal of Development Studies* 50(10):1397–1410.

Thomas SL, Wakerman J, Humphreys JS. (2015) Ensuring equity of access to primary health care in rural and remote Australia – What core services should be locally available? *International Journal for Equity in Health* 14(111):1–8.

Thomson K, Hillier-Brown F, Todd A, McNamara C, Huijts T, Bambra C. (2018) The effects of public health policies on health inequalities in high-income countries: An umbrella review. *BMC Public Health* 18(869):1–21.

Tirgil A, Gurol-Urganci I, Atun R. (2018) Early experience of universal health coverage in Turkey on access to health services for the poor: Regression kink design analysis. *Journal of Global Health* 8(2):1–9.

Torbica A, Tarricone R, Drummond M. (2018) Does the approach to economic evaluation in health care depend on culture, values, and institutional context? *The European Journal of Health Economics* 19(6):769–774.

Tyebjee T, Hardin J. (2004) Biotech-pharma alliances: Strategies, structures and financing. *Journal of Commercial Biotechnology* 10(4):329–339.

Van Doorslaer E, Koolman X, Jones AM. (2004) Explaining income-related inequalities in doctor utilisation in Europe. *Health Economics* 13(7):629–647.

Van Doorslaer E, Wagstaff A, Calonge S, Christiansen T, Gerfin M, Gottschalk P, Janssen R, Lachaud C, Leu RE, Nolan B, et al. (1992) Equity in the delivery of health care: Some international comparisons. *Journal of Health Economics* 11(4):389–411.

Varabyova Y, Schreyögg J. (2013) International comparisons of the technical efficiency of the hospital sector: Panel data analysis of OECD countries using parametric and non-parametric approach. *Health Policy* 112(1–2):70–79.

Wade RH. (2004) Is globalization reducing poverty and inequality? *International Journal of Health Services* 34(3):381–414.

Wagstaff A, van Doorslaer E. (2000) *Equity in health care finance and delivery*. InI North Holland Handbook in Health Economics, ed. A. Culyer and J. Newhouse, 1804–1862. North Holland: Amsterdam, Netherlands.

Wagstaff A. (2002). Poverty and health sector inequalities. *Bulletin of the World Health Organization* 80(2):97–105.

Wensing M, Grol R. (2019) Knowledge translation in health: How implementation science could contribute more. *BMC Medicine* 17(88):1–6.

Whitehead M. (1992) The concepts and principles of equity and health. *International Journal of Health Services* 22(3):429–445.

World Bank (WB) (2014) Turkey's transition, integration, inclusion, institutions. The WB International Bank for Reconstruction and Development. Washington, D.C.

World Bank (WB). (2019) World Bank Country and Lending Groups. https:// datahelpdesk.worldbank.org/knowledgebase/articles/906519-world-bank-country-and-lending-groups. Accessed on: 1.4.2019.

World Health Organization (WHO). (1981) Global Strategy for Health for All by the Year 2000. Geneva, Switzerland.

World Health Organization (WHO). (2006) Working together for health. The World Health Report, Geneva, Switzerland.

World Health Organization (WHO). (2008) Closing the Gap in a Generation: Generation Health Equity Through Action on the Social Determinants of Health: Commission on Social Determinants of Health Final Report. Geneva. www.who.int/social_determinants/thecommission/en/. Accessed on: 1.5.2019.

World Health Organization (WHO). (2013a) Closing the health equity gap. Policy options and opportunities for action. World Health Organization. WHO Library Cataloguing-in Publication Data. Geneva, Switzerland.

World Health Organization (WHO). (2013b) Handbook on health inequality monitoring with a special focus on low- and middle-income countries. https:// apps.who.int/iris/bitstream/handle/10665/85345/9789241548632_eng.pdf;jse ssionid=0EDEC1104741952EFEF7CB6B129EB295?sequence=1. Accessed on: 27.2.2019.

World Health Organization (WHO). (2016) Social Determinants of Health. World Health Organization. www.who.int/social_determinants/en/. Accessed on: 1.8.2017.

World Health Organization (WHO)-Declaration of Alma-Ata. (1978) Alma-Ata: International Conference on Primary Health Care www.who.int/publications/ almaata_declaration_en.pdf. Accessed on: 9.9.2015.

Xu K, Klavus J, Aguilar-Rivera AM, Carrin G, Zeramdini R, Murray CJL. (2003) Summary measures of the distribution of household financial contributions to health. Health Systems Performance Assessment, Murray C.L., Evans D.B. (eds) (Chapter 40). WHO: Geneva, pp. 543–555.

Xu K, Saksena P, Holly A. (2011) The determinants of health expenditure. A Country-Country Level Panel Data Analysis. Analysis WHO. www.who.int/health_finan-cing/documents/report_en_11_deter-he.pdf?ua=1. Accessed on: 22.2.2019.

Yardim MS, Çilingiroğlu N, Yardim N. (2014) Financial protection in health in Turkey: The effects of the Health Transformation Programme. *Health Policy and Planning* 29(2):177–192.

Zelman WN, Pink GH, Matthias CB. (2003) Using balanced scorecard in health care. *Journal of Health Care Finance* 29(4):1–16.

Zheng H. (2012) Do people die from income inequality of a decade ago? *Social Science & Medicine* 75(1):36–45.

Chapter 2

International comparison of equity in healthcare services

The level of equity in healthcare services is one of the primary performance measures in healthcare (Kruk and Freedman, 2008). In other words, it is possible to compare international health systems by considering the level of equity for different health functions.

Studying the distribution of health expenditures in terms of income differences is a traditional way of international equity analysis in healthcare. However, the design of the health system (Wong et al., 2015), priorities of health policymakers regarding resource distribution (Sheldon and Smith, 2000), political factors and health reform experiences (Janes et al., 2006), country development level (Wagstaff et al., 1989), sociodemographic (Kirst et al., 2013) and cultural (Corona et al., 2019) factors are strong determinants of cross-country differences in health equities.

This book chapter focuses on international comparison of equity in healthcare services. In this regard, firstly, a summary will be given about international differences in the level of health expenditures. After that, international differences regarding the concern for equity is explained. Subsequently, the interrelationship between health reforms and health equity is mentioned with a discussion regarding current health system problems and imminent need to consider equity in healthcare.

International comparison of equity in healthcare services

International comparison of healthcare system performance is an essential task for health policymakers (Varabyova and Schreyögg, 2013). Analysis of the level of equity in the distribution of healthcare expenditures and healthcare-service use allows analysts to examine the degree of fairness of distribution of healthcare expenditure and healthcare services. Ensuring an equal distribution of healthcare services by considering the benefits and values of individuals is a type of healthcare system performance measure (Alberti et al., 2013). The decisions of policymakers from developed countries are in line with the definition of "equity," and they suggest that payments toward healthcare should be related to the ability to pay rather than to the use of medical facilities (Wagstaff and van Doorslaer, 1992).

The pattern of the distribution of out-of-pocket (OOP) health expenses and different functions of health services have garnered the interest of health policymakers in different countries (Haakenstad et al., 2019). The distinguishing feature of the distributive pattern of OOP health expenses in developed countries is its regressive pattern. In other words, the financial burden of OOP health expenditures falls on the shoulders of poor households (Wagstaff et al., 1989). This statement can be clarified further using the literature that shows that the Netherlands, Britain, and the US were found to have a regressive financing system. Among these countries, Britain has a mildly progressive financing system. The Dutch system was marginally less regressive than the American system. Specifically, the US has a regressive system (Wagstaff et al., 1989).

An updated study regarding the distributional implications of alternative healthcare financing reforms in European countries and the US shows that the total healthcare payments are almost proportional to the ability to pay in most countries. Moreover, private payments – OOP payments as well as private insurance premiums – are highly regressive. Notably, private payments put a heavy burden on unfortunate households (De Graeve and van Ourti, 2003).

Equity analysis of the distributive pattern of OOP health expenses necessitates detailed methodological analysis. Obviously, international comparison of equity analysis is a multidisciplinary field of research. Several studies exist in the literature regarding the comparison of different index scores by using the same dataset or incorporating quantitative analysis tools, such as Monte Carlo simulations, weighting procedures, optimization techniques, etc. In this regard, equity analysis in healthcare is a multidimensional field of research (Ivaldi et al., 2016; Erreygers et al., 2012; Dufour et al., 2017; Atems and Shand, 2018; Karagrigoriou et al., 2018).

International differences in the level of health expenditures

Traditionally, most studies related to equity in the delivery of healthcare conducted in European countries and the US gave more importance to the distribution of welfare (Beckfield et al., 2015). Developed country experiences have stated that healthcare should be distributed according to the need rather than the willingness or ability to pay (Fein, 2005).

Organization for Economic Co-operation and Development (OECD) countries are specific examples of developed nations. Most of the members of OECD countries are from Europe and currently spend high amounts on healthcare (Huber and Orozs, 2003). In these countries, the health -care system constitutes the largest service industry with the average health expenditure reaching 9.5% of the GDP in 2010 (Varabyova and Schreyögg, 2013).

Pharmaceutical expenditures constitute a major part of health expenditures. There is more evident inequity in the distribution of pharmaceutical expenses in the US. The US represents an extreme example among the OECD countries because of the high level of expenditures on health (OECD, 2017). However, the US is the leader in research and development of innovative health technologies, such as the pharmaceutical sector. High costs undoubtedly increase the level of pharmaceutical expenditures and create differences in health expenditure (Papanicolas et al., 2018).

The US has much higher total expenditure as a share of its economy and its public health expenditures alone are in line with other developed countries. For instance, the private expenditure in the US is much higher at 8.8% of GDP compared with any other country, which is at 2.7% on average (OECD, 2019). Supportive evidence comes from the literature and emphasizes that the US spends more per capita on healthcare than any other country. Moreover, private health expenditure ranges between 15% and 30% of the total healthcare expenditure in OECD countries (Del Vecchio et al., 2015).

The gap regarding health expenditure between the US and other comparable countries has widened in recent years. Figure 2.1 shows health expenditure in OECD countries and the US for the year 2017. Therefore, the US is undoubtedly the leader in terms of health expenditure among the OECD countries (OECD, 2019).

The level of health expenditures reflects the health outcomes and determines the level of equity in health resources distribution (Marmot et al., 2007). Figure 2.2 shows that in all the OECD countries both the life expectancy at birth and health expenditure have increased over time. However,

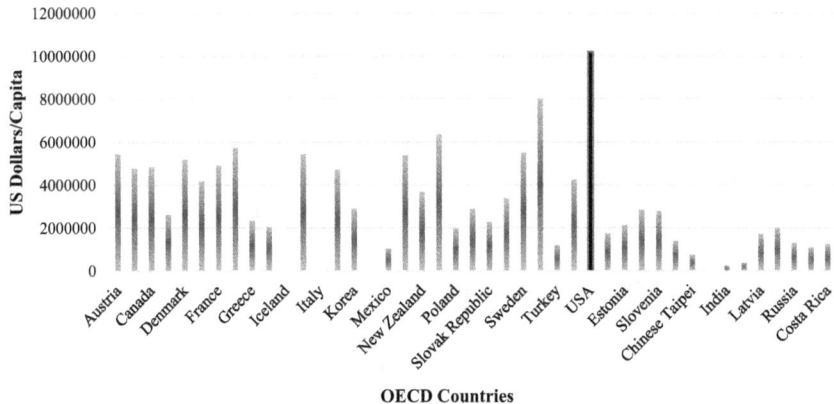

Figure 2.1 Health spending in OECD countries and in the US.

Source: OECD Data Health Spending, Health expenditure and financing, Total/ Government/compulsory / Voluntary, US dollars/capita, 2017 or latest available. Retrieved from: https://data.oecd.org/healthres/health-spending.htm. Accessed on: 24.1.2019.

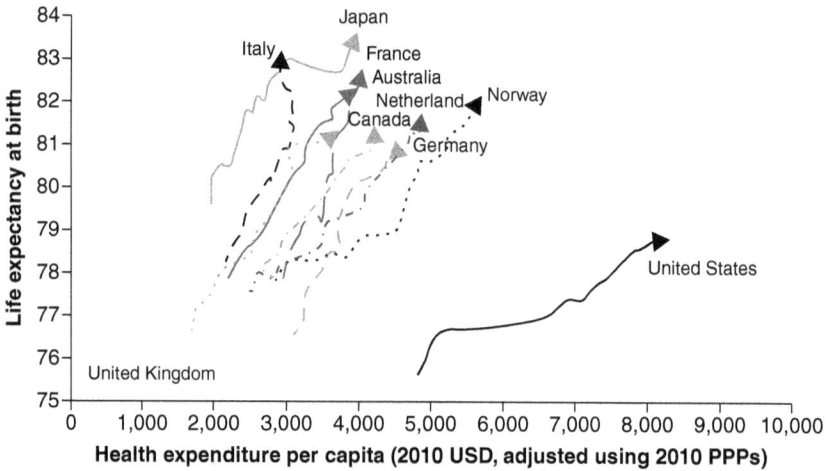

Figure 2.2 Life expectancy gains and increased health spending, selected high income countries, 1995–2015.

Source: OECD Indicators Health at a Glance, 2017: OECD Indicators, OECD Publishing, Paris.
Retrieved from: http://dx.doi.org/10.1787/health_glance-2017-en. Accessed on: 24.3.2019.

the level of increase is not the same in all OECD countries. The US is an
outlier, and its life expectancy gains have been smaller. On the other hand,
Japan is the leader in life expectancy gains and has reached almost 84 years
between 1995 and 2015. However, Japan's level of health expenditure per
capita is smaller than that of the US despite the increase in the health status
of the population (OECD, 2017). Based on these indicators, the efficient
use of health resources and health expenditure is a dubious issue for most
of the developed economies. In other words, increasing the level of health
expenses reflects little into the health status of the population in developed
economies such as in the US, financial burden of medical care are borne by
poor Americans (Dickman et al., 2017). A little reflection of the increase in
health expenses on health outcomes brings on to the table the concern of
efficient management of health resources (Cylus et al., 2016).

International differences regarding the concern for equity

The inefficient use of financial resources in healthcare mandates an
assessment of the situation from the equity perspective (Whitehead et al.,
2001). Literature ascertains that there is a strong interrelationship between
equity and efficiency. However, there is a lack of empirical evidence regarding
whether an increase in equity results in a decrease in efficiency (Karsu and
Morton, 2015). An answer to this question and detailed examination of
the interrelationship between equity and efficiency will prove significantly

beneficial for developing and underdeveloped countries owing to the financial resource constraints (Blank, 2002; Karsu and Morton, 2015).

Equal distribution of welfare is one of the primary concerns of equity analysis. However, the degree of the distribution of equity is not the same for all developed nations (Ortiz and Cummins, 2011). The vulnerable groups living in developed nations undoubtedly are at a disadvantage because of the unequal distribution of resources. Moreover, the literature suggests that in the developed world, the single most reliable predictor of an individual's health is his/her position in the socioeconomic spectrum (Lal et al., 2018).

This statement can be clarified by reviewing a study that compared inequalities in the health of five nations: Australia, Canada, New Zealand, the UK, and the US. The study results showed that low-income US citizens reported more problems accessing care than their counterparts in the other four countries (Blendon et al., 2002).

Building and improving the capacity to ensure equal distribution of health resources takes precedence for global health leadership organizations, such as The WHO (WHO, 2013). WHO developed a toolkit for the assessment of health inequalities in different countries. Health Equity Assessment Toolkit (HEAT) is a software application that represents health inequalities within countries. HEAT system allows users to upload their databases and assess inequalities in this system. HEAT is open-source software and operates on Windows and Macintosh platforms and is downloadable from the WHO website. This system enables the monitoring of global and national inequality assessments. Further developments in this system will include interactive graphs, which will be translated into different languages (Hosseinpoor et al., 2018).

HEAT Plus is a flexible method, and this makes it a good alternative for the analysis of global health equity. It is necessary to point out that developed European countries have better technology and leadership in pharmaceutical technologies. Therefore, ensuring a collaborative atmosphere between developed and developing countries will prove beneficial in improving global health with consideration of equality (Pratt and Hyder, 2016).

Horizontal equity in the utilization of healthcare services has also been evaluated using evidence from Asian economies. Study results show that there is prowealth inequity in Western countries regarding doctor visits, whereas Taiwan is either proportional or slightly the opposite (Lu et al., 2007).

Developing countries face specific situations to ensure equity in healthcare services. Recent reports reveal that 93% of the global burden of preventable mortality occurs in developing countries; however, there is negligible funding for the research and resolution of healthcare problems in developing countries (Sitthi-amorn and Somrongthong, 2000).

Distribution of health resources and the degree of health transfers is different in developing countries. In other words, rural and urban differences are more apparent in developing countries that have emerging economies

(Fotso, 2006). Therefore, unequal distribution of resources and welfare state make accessibility of healthcare services and utilization of healthcare difficult, and the poor people are at a disadvantage. Notably, the international differences in socially inclusive policies will influence the welfare distribution of populations (Thomson et al., 2016).

China is a specific example of an emerging economy country, and several researchers in the field of health equity analysis have questioned the amount of social inclusiveness (Deng et al., 2013). More than a decade ago, the Chinese government had committed to increasing government finance for healthcare by directing 1%–%–1.5% of GDP to universal basic healthcare services. Notably, the total health expenditure and total pharmaceutical expenditure have increased rapidly in China over the past few decades. Drug expenditure makes up to 2.28% of total GDP, and this trend is much higher than the OECD average of 1.5% (OECD, 2013; NHDRC, 2013; Hu and Mossialos, 2016). Consequently, the pharmaceutical expenditure/total health expenditure is higher than that of Brazil (~12%), Russia (~18%), or India (~26%) (McKinsey & Company, 2020; Deloitte, 2015; BMI Research, 2015).

A high amount of resource allocation into healthcare mandates questioning of the efficiency of health system regulations (Kruk and Pate, 2020). Preliminary analysis results have stated that because of cost inflation and wasteful healthcare delivery system, the Chinese health system is inefficient, and a vast amount of money is likely pocketed as higher income and profits by the providers (Yip and Hsiao, 2008).

China's health system reform can provide lessons for developing countries. China successfully achieved universal health coverage in 2011 – the most massive expansion of insurance coverage in human history. Notably, more than 95% of the Chinese population is insured under this universal coverage, and most importantly, this increase in health coverage includes both the rural and urban population. According to the National Health Services Survey for the years 1998, 2003, and 2008, population coverage of health insurance schemes by rural and urban areas are presented in Figure 2.3.

This high proportion of universal health coverage has garnered the interest of political and social analysts, and they have provided a brief overview of the underlying factors that led to the successful high-degree universal health coverage in China (Meng et al., 2015). Strong political support for government intervention in healthcare, renewed political commitment from top leaders, heavy government subsidies, and a strong capacity based on China's economic power are the factors behind China's success in achieving universal health coverage (Qingyue and Shenglan, 2013; Yu, 2015).

Health reforms and health equity

Ensuring a more socially inclusive health system is one of the primary motivations of global health system reforms with the developing

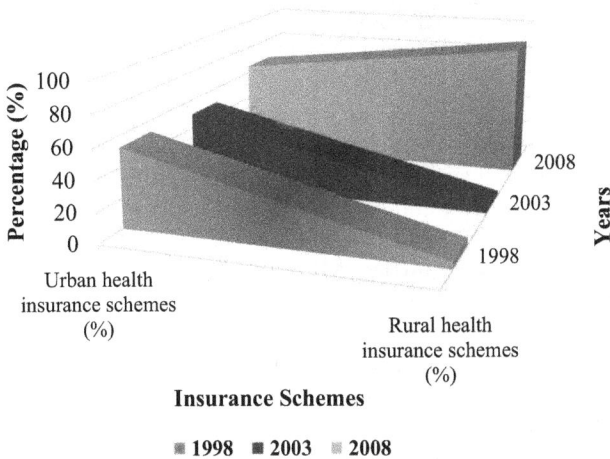

Figure 2.3 Population coverage of health insurance schemes by urban and rural areas in China, 1998–2008.

Sources: Modified from National Health Services Survey 1998, 2003, and 2008

countries showing a more obvious motivation because of the scarcity of financial and other resources (Gupta and Vegelin, 2016). Thus, ensuring an equitable health system and an equal redistribution of health and medical technologies are the main principles of health system regulations (WHO, 2013).

Latin American countries that represent developing countries started social sector reforms in the 1980s to reduce socioeconomic inequalities, improve health outcomes, and provide financial risk protection (de Andrade et al., 2015). The focus of health system reforms that began in 1990 was to primarily decrease inequalities and improve health outcomes while focusing on universal health coverage. The primary concern was protecting the poor citizens (Atun et al., 2015). Notably, unequal societies characterize Latin American countries. However, poverty has shown a decreasing trend in Latin American and Caribbean countries. Notably, the poverty rate in Latin America and the Caribbean was 43.3% in 2000, and this has decreased to 24.6% in 2016 (WB, 2018).

In Latin America, the total drug expenditures in 2003 amounted to approximately $19 billion. Countries in the region spend between 7% and 16% of their public health sector budgets on pharmaceuticals: 16% in Argentina, 7.7% in Costa Rica, 8.3% in Honduras, 15.2% in Venezuela, and, excluding the social security institute, 9.4% in the Dominican Republic. As in the other parts of the world, the cost of medicines is increasing at a faster rate than the other health services, and pharmaceuticals are the highest OOP health expenditure for the poor (Homedes et al., 2005).

A considerable amount of inequity is observed in Latin American countries. A survey of seven Latin American countries reported that the lowest income quintile allocated 52% of all health expenditures to drugs, whereas for the highest income quintile, drugs represented 30% of their health expenditures (Pan American Health Organization, 2012).

The effect of socially inclusive policies regarding health expenditures on the level of equity is primarily significant for underdeveloped African countries. The existing literature reveals a regressive pattern of the distribution of health expenses in African countries (Mills et al., 2012).

The contribution of social health insurance on health insurance is questionable, and it has been stated that the introduction of the scheme will reduce potential differences between benefit packages (Kerssens and Groenewegen, 2005). However, this will help to solve inequity problems existing among civil servants, but not the entire country. Therefore, even though social insurance can benefit civil servants, it may not provide benefits to the whole community (Goudge et al., 2018).

Current health system problems and increasing need to consider equity in health

International comparison of health system inequities warrants awareness of current trends in healthcare. In this regard, one of the well-known healthcare management thinkers, Mintzberg (2017), makes a very brief overview of the current health system problems (Adinolfi and Borgonovi, 2018).

One of these problems is related to the wrong belief that health systems are failing. This incorrect interpretation is because of the failure to understand real health system problems and provide temporary solutions (Adinolfi and Borgonovi, 2018). The second problem is related to the lack of a point of view regarding multidimensional and comprehensive solutions. Mintzberg (2017) advises using a social engineering perspective into the solution of health system problems, and this will necessitate incorporating different stakeholders and the community into the healthcare decision-making processes. The third myth emphasizes the role of strong leadership to improve the long-term effects of health reforms. This is the primary concern of health policymakers in developed and developing countries. This myth highlights that international health system problems can be fixed, if it is treated more like a business. The reason behind this statement is to strengthen competition in the private health sector (Adinolfi and Borgonovi, 2018).

The US is a specific example of a country that prioritizes private sector and supports competitive health market. This health system policy brings pros and cons on to the table. Notably, the US spends considerably more on health compared with other developed countries (Papanicolas et al., 2008). Moreover, the poor population of the US is faced with problems regarding the health insurance system and lack of social inclusiveness. However, high expenditure on new health technologies, such as drug development and pharmaceuticals and advanced treatments, makes the US the leader in research and development in healthcare (Murthy and Okunade, 2016).

The final myth of Mintzberg (2018) is related to the main difference between the public and private sectors in healthcare. Traditionally, it is believed that the public sector is controlled for the sake of equality, whereas the private sector operates for the sake of efficiency. Even though considering a balance between these two principal health system dynamics is essential for the sustainability of every health system, the degree of importance given to each of these dynamics is different (Adinolfi and Borgonovi, 2018).

Mintzberg (2018) advises public managers to be more aware of improving efficiencies in health systems (Adinolfi and Borgonovi, 2018). Additionally, this will necessitate incorporating private sector management tools and strategies into the public health system. The competitive pharmaceutical market can provide many insights and include several private sector-oriented models to improve the efficiency of health services (Vicente and Simoes, 2014).

Public–private partnership (PPP) models are one of the current public management strategies to enable collaboration between the public and private sectors (Meissner, 2019). This strategy will prove beneficial for the private sector expertise. According to the report prepared by European PPP expertise, Turkey, Italy, and the United Kingdom are the leading countries in terms of the value of PPP projects and the number of projects in 2014. Education, health, and transportation are common areas that are used in PPP models (EPEC, 2017).

Increasing the number of PPP projects in healthcare necessitates questioning of equal distribution of resources in healthcare (Torchia et al., 2015). Thus, considering a perfect balance when distributing resources between public and private systems is essential for the future sustainability of healthcare systems. To conclude, the changing nature of global health system dynamics and inclusion of private sector more into the health system increases competition in the pharmaceutical market and causes higher health expenditures, thereby bringing equity dynamics on to the table (Danzon, 2018).

The health insurance market design provides more benefits to the private sector. Private and complementary health insurance markets have strong growth potential globally (Preker et al., 2010). Notably, developing countries are using public funding to function their health systems. In other words, the government directly provides and finances health system payments. However, this system is not sustainable and fails to provide adequate financial protection for the vulnerable groups. Limitations of the public system necessitate financial support, which is possible with the incorporation of the private sector into the system (Pauly et al., 2006).

Overall, considering the myths of the health system and providing permanent solutions to these problems is necessary to ensure equity in the health systems of developed and developing countries (Adinolfi and Borgonovi, 2018). To conclude, it is essential to understand the main structure of private healthcare expenditure and consider equity in the distribution of healthcare expenditures by focusing on costly areas of health services, such as pharmaceutical expenditures. To sum up, further monitoring of inequalities is essential to assess whether equality is being considered in income and healthcare service distribution regularly. Following chapters of this book provides an overview about equity in the distribution of health services in developing countries and close look at equity lessons learned from pharmerging countries, which are experiencing health reforms.

References

Adinolfi P, Borgonovi E. (2018) *The myths of health care. Towards New Models of Leadership and Management in the Healthcare Sector*. Foreword by Henry Mintzberg. Springer International Publishing AG: Switzerland.

Alberti PM, Bonham AC, Kirch DG. (2013) Making equity a value in value-based health care. *Academic Medicine* 88(11):1619–1623.

Atems B, Shand G. (2018) An empirical analysis of the relationship between entrepreneurship and income inequality. *Small Business Economics* 51(4):905–922.

Atun R, de Andrade LOM, Almeida G, Cotlear D, Dmytraczenko T, Frenz P, Garcia P, Gómez-Dantés, O. Knaul FM, Muntaner C, Braga de Paula J, Rígoli F, Castell-Florit Serrate P. Wagstaff A. (2015) Health system reform and universal health coverage in Latin America. *The Lancet* 385(9974):1230–1247.

Beckfield J, Bambra C, Eikemo TA, Huijts T, McNamara C, Wendt C. (2015) An institutional theory of welfare state effects on the distribution of population health. *Social Theory & Health* 13(3/4):227–244.

Blank RM. (2002) Can equity and efficiency complement each other? *Labour Economics* 9(4):451–468.

Blendon RJ, Schoen C, DesRoches CM, Osborn R, Scoles KL, Zapert K. (2002) Inequities in health care: A five-country survey. *Health Affairs* (Millwood) 21(3):182–191.

BMI Research. (2015) Russia Pharmaceuticals & Healthcare Report; *2015*. London.

China National Health Services Survey. 1998, 2003 and 2008. National Bureau of Statistics of China. http://www.stats.gov.cn/english/.

Corona K, Campos B, Rook KS, Biegler K, Sorkin DH (2019) Do cultural values have a role in health equity? A study of Latina mothers and daughters. *Cultural Diversity and Ethnic Minority Psychology* 25(1):65–72.

Cylus J, Papanicolas I, Smith PC. (2016) Health system efficiency: How to make measurement matter for policy and management. European Observatory on Health Systems and Policies. Chapter 7. Cylus J, Pearson M. Cross-national efficiency comparisons of health systems, subsectors and disease areas, pp. 139–164. www.euro.who.int/__data/assets/pdf_file/0004/324283/Health-System-Efficiency-How-make-measurement-matter-policy-management.pdf. Accessed on: 8.2.2020.

Danzon PM. (2018) Differential pricing of pharmaceuticals: Theory, evidence and emerging issues. *PharmacoEconomics* 36(12):1395–1405.

de Andrade LOM, Pellegrini Filho A, Solar O, Rígoli F, de Salazar LM, Serrate PC, Ribeiro KG, Koller TS, Cruz FN, Atun R. (2015) Social determinants of health, universal health coverage, and sustainable development: Case studies from Latin American countries. *The Lancet* 385(9975):1343–1351.

de Graeve D, van Ourti (2003) The distributional impact of health financing in Europe: A review. *The World Economy* 26(10):1459–1479.

Del Vecchio MD, Fenech L, Prenestini A. (2015) Private health care expenditure and quality in Beveridge systems: Cross-regional differences in the Italian NHS. *Health Policy* 119(3):356–366.

Deloitte. (2015) 2015 life sciences outlook Brazil; 2015. Sao Paulo. www2.deloitte. com/content/dam/Deloitte/global/Documents/Life-Sciences-Healthcare/gx-lshc-2015-life-sciences-report-brazil.pdf. Accessed on: 20.2.2019.

Deng S, Sherraden M, Huang J, Jin M. (2013) Asset opportunity for the poor: An asset-based policy agenda towards inclusive growth in China. *China Journal of Social Work* 6(1):40–51.

Dickman SL, Himmelstein DU, Woolhandler S. (2017) Inequality and the health-care system in the USA. *The Lancet* 389(10077):1431–1441.

Dufour JM, Flachaire E, Khalaf L. (2017) Permutation tests for comparing inequality measures. *Journal of Business & Economic Statistics* 37(3):457–470.

Erreygers G, Clarke P, van Ourti T. (2012) "Mirror, mirror, on the wall, who in this land is the fairest of all?" – Distributional sensitivity in the measurement of socio-economic inequality of health. *Journal of Health Economics* 31(1):257–270.

European PPP Expertise Center (EPEC). (2017) Market Update Review of the European PPP Market in 2017. www.eib.org/attachments/epec/epec_market_update_2017_en.pdf. Accessed on: 23.2.2019.

Fein R. (2005) On achieving access and equity in health care. *The Milbank Quarterly* 83(4):1–35.

Fotso JC. (2006) Child health inequities in developing countries: Differences across urban and rural areas. *International Journal for Equity in Health* 5(9):1–10.

Goudge J, Alaba OA, Govender V, Harris B, Nxumalo N, Chersich MF. (2018) Social health insurance contributes to universal coverage in South Africa, but generates inequities: Survey among members of a government employee insurance scheme. *International Journal for Equity in Health* 17(1):1–13.

Gupta J, Vegelin C. (2016) Sustainable development goals and inclusive development. International Environmental Agreements: Politics, *Law and Economics* 16:433–448.

Haakenstad A, Coates M, Marx A, Bukhman G, Verguet S. (2019) Disaggregating catastrophic health expenditure by disease area: Cross-country estimates based on the World Health Surveys. *BMC Medicine* 17(36):1–9.

Homedes N, Ugalde A, Forns JR. (2005) The World Bank, pharmaceutical policies, and health reforms in Latin America. *International Journal of Health Services* 35(4):691–717.

Hosseinpoor AR, Schlotgheuber A, Nambiar D, Ross Z. (2018) Health equity assessment toolkit plus (HEAT Plus): Software for exploring and comparing health inequalities using uploaded datasets. *Global Health Action* 11:20–30.

Hu J, Mossialos E. (2016) Pharmaceutical pricing and reimbursement in China: When the whole is less than the sum of its parts. *Health Policy* 120(5):519–534.

Huber M, Orosz E. (2003) Health expenditure trends in OECD countries, 1990–2001. *Health Care Financing Review* 25(1):1–22.

Ivaldi E, Bonatti G, Soliani R. (2016) The construction of a synthetic index comparing multidimensional well-being in the European Union. *Social Indicators Research* 125(2):397–430.

Janes CR, Chuluundorj O, Hilliard CE, Rak K, Janchiv K. (2006) Poor medicine for poor people? Assessing the impact of neoliberal reform on health care equity in a post-socialist context. *Global Public Health* 1(1):5–30.

Karagrigoriou A, Makrides A, Vonta I. (2018) On a control chart for the Gini index with simulations. *Communications in Statistics-Simulation and Computation* 48(4):1121–1137.

Karsu Ö, Morton A. (2015) Inequity averse optimization in operational research. *European Journal of Operational Research* 245(2):343–359.

Kerssens JJ. Groenewegen PP. (2005) Consumer preferences in social health insurance. *The European Journal of Health Economics* 50:8–15.

Kirst M, Shankardass K, Bomse S, Lofters A, Quiñonez C. (2013) Sociodemographic data collection for health equity measurement: A mixed methods study examining public opinions. *International Journal for Equity in Health* 12(75):1–10.

Kruk ME, Freedman LP. (2008) Assessing health system performance in developing countries: A review of the literature. *Health Policy* 85(3):263–276.

Kruk ME, Pate M. (2020) The lancet global health commission on high quality health systems 1 year on: Progress on a global imperative. *The Lancet* 8(1):e30–e32.

Lal A, Moodie M, Peeters A, Carter R. (2018) Inclusion of equity in economic analyses of public health policies: Systematic review and future directions. *Australian and New Zealand Journal of Public Health* 42(2):207–213.

Lu JR, Leung GM, Kwon S, Tin KY, van Doorslaer E, O'Donnell O. (2007). Horizontal equity in health care utilization evidence from three high-income Asian economies. *Social Science & Medicine* 64(1):199–212.

Marmot M. (2007) Achieving health equity: From root causes to fair outcomes. *The Lancet* 370(9593):1153–1163.

McKinsey & Company. India Pharma. (2020). Propelling access and acceptance, realising true potential. Pharmaceutical and Medical Products Practice. http://online.wsj.com/public/resources/documents/McKinseyPharma2020ExecutiveSummary.pdf. Accessed on: 20.2.2019.

Meissner D. (2019) Public-private partnership models for science, technology, and innovation cooperation. *Journal of the Knowledge Economy* 10:1341–1361.

Meng Q, Fang H, Liu X, Yuan B, Xu J. (2015) Consolidating the social health insurance schemes in China: Towards an equitable and efficient health system. *The Lancet* 386(10002):1484–1492.

Mills A, Ataguba JE, Akazili J, Borghi J, Garshong B, Makawia S, Mtei G, Harris B, Macha J, Meheus F, McIntyre D. (2012) Equity in financing and use of health care in Ghana, South Africa, and Tanzania: Implications for paths to universal Coverage. *The Lancet* 380(9837):126–133.

Mintzberg, H. (2017) *Managing the myths of health care: Bridging the seperations between care, cure, control and community*. Berrett-Koehler Publishers, Inc. Oakland, CA.

Murthy VNR, Okunade AA. (2016) Determinants of U.S. health expenditure: Evidence from autoregressive distributed lag (ARDL) approach to cointegration. *Economic Modelling* 59:67–73.

National Health Development Research Center. (NHDRC) (2013) China National Health Accounts Report. Beijing.

Organization for Economic Co-operation and Development (OECD). (2013) Health at a glance 2013 – OECD indicators; 2013. Paris. www.oecd.org/els/health-systems/Health-at-a-Glance-2013.pdf. Accessed on: 20.2.2019.

Organization for Economic Co-operation and Development (OECD). (2017) Data health spending, Health expenditure and financing, Total/ Government/compulsory / Voluntary, US dollars/capita, 2017 or latest available. https://data.oecd.org/healthres/health-spending.htm. Accessed on: 24.1.2019.

Organization for Economic Co-operation and Development (OECD). (2019) https://data.oecd.org/healthres/health-spending.htm. Accessed on: 20.2.2019.

Ortiz I, Cummins M. (2011) Global inequality: Beyond the bottom billion – a rapid review of income distribution in 141 countries. https://ssrn.com/abstract=1805046 or http://dx.doi.org/10.2139/ssrn.1805046. Accessed on: 28.2.2020.

Pan American Health Organization. (2012). Health Care Expenditure and Financing in Latin America and the Caribbean. [Fact Sheet]. prepared by Rubén M. Suárez-Berenguela and William Vigil-Oliver. Area of Health Systems Based on Primary Health Care Pan America Health Organization/World Health Organization (PAHO/WHO). Washington, D.C.

Papanicolas I, Woskie LR, Jha AK. (2018) Health care spending in the United States and other high-income countries. *JAMA* 319(10):1024–1039.

Pauly MV, Zweifel P, Scheffler RM, Preker AS, Bassett M. (2006) Private health insurance in developing countries. *Health Affairs* (Millwood) 25(2):369–379.

Pratt B, Hyder AA. (2016) Governance of transnational global health research consortia and health equity. *The American Journal of Bioethics* 16(10):29–45.

Preker AS, Zweifel P, Schellekens O. (2010) *Global marketplace for private health insurance: Strength in numbers*. The World Bank: Washington, D.C. https://doi.org/10.1596/978-0-8213-7507-5.

Qingyue M, Shenglan T. (2013) Universal health care coverage in China: Challenges and opportunities. *Procedia – Social and Behavioral Sciences* 77:330–340.

Sheldon TA, Smith PC. (2000) Equity in the allocation of health care resources. *Health Economics* 9(7):571–574.

Sitthi-amorn C, Somrongthong R. (2000) Strengthening health research capacity in developing countries: A critical element for achieving health equity. *British Medical Journal* 321(7264):813–817.

The World Bank. (2018) LAC Equity Lab: Poverty – Poverty Rate. www.worldbank.org/en/topic/poverty/lac-equity-lab1/poverty/head-count. Accessed on: 20.2.2019.

Thomson K, Bambra C, McNamara C, Huijts T, Todd A. (2016) The effects of public health policies on population health and health inequalities in European welfare states: Protocol for an umbrella review. *Systematic Reviews* 5:57. https://doi.org/10.1186/s13643-016-0235-3.

Torchia M, Calabró A, Morner M. (2015) Public–private partnerships in the health care sector: Asystematic review of the literature. *Public Management Review* 17(2):236–261.

Varabyova Y, Schreyögg J. (2013) International comparisons of the technical efficiency of the hospital sector: Panel data analysis of OECD countries using parametric and non-parametric approaches. *Health Policy* 112(1–2):70–79.

Vicente V, Simóes S. (2014) Manufacturing and export provisions: Impact on the competitiveness of European pharmaceutical manufacturers and on the creation of jobs in Europe. *Journal of Generic Medicines: The Business Journal for the Generic Medicines Sector* 11(1–2):35–47.

Wagstaff A, van Doorslaer E, Calonge S, Christiansen T, Gerfin M, Gottschalk P, Janssen R, Lachaud C, Leu RE, Nolan B. et al. (1992) Equity in the finance of health care: Some international comparisons. *Journal of Health Economics* 11(4):361–387.

Wagstaff A, van Doorslaer E, Paci P. (1989) Equity in the finance and delivery of health care: Some tentative cross-country comparisons. *Oxford Review of Economic Policy* 5(1):89–112.

Whitehead M. Dahlgren G. Evans T. (2001) Equity and health sector reforms: Can low-income countries escape the medical poverty trap? *The Lancet* 358(9284): 833–836.

Wong WF, LaVeist TA, Sharfstein JM. (2015) Achieving health equity by design. *JAMA* 313(14):1417–1418.

World Health Organization (WHO). (2013) Handbook on health inequality monitoring. with a special focus on low- and middle-income countries. https://apps.who.int/iris/bitstream/handle/10665/85345/9789241548632_eng.pdf?sequence=1. Accessed on: 26.2.2020.

Yip W, Hsiao WC. (2008) The Chinese health system at a crossroads. *Health Affairs* (Millwood) 27(2):460–468.

Yu H. (2015) Universal health insurance coverage for 1.3 billion people: What accounts for China's success? *Health Policy* 119(9):1145–1152.

Chapter 3

Equity in health services and policy advice for developing countries

Developing countries have failed to provide and sustain financial access to high-quality healthcare services. Increases in government expenditures to strengthen the primary healthcare system are priority strategies to provide healthcare equity in developing countries (Tangcharoensathien et al., 2015). Most developing countries have highly competitive pharmaceutical markets; they are known as "pharmerging" countries. In these countries, healthcare equity is poor because the research capacity of these countries is weaker than that of developed nations (Mitsumori, 2019). Thus, the gap in health equity is widening between and within countries. Strengthening health research capacity in developing countries is a way to achieve health equity in developing countries (Sitthi-amorn and Somrongthong, 2000). To fight against inequities in healthcare, strong cooperation between developed and developing countries and a global commitment to improve equity are essential (Sitthi-amorn and Somrongthong, 2000).

Strong political commitment to increase fiscal capacity can help provide equity in financial resource distribution for less-developed countries (Tangcharoensathien et al., 2015). Comprehensive and inclusive health policies will improve global health. Increased cooperation among professionals from different fields of healthcare, both medical and nonmedical, is necessary to achieve better global health (Schmitt et al., 2011). Strong primary care will improve public health and improve population health status in developing countries. (Lee et al., 2007).

A systemwide approach must be established for better management of global health and to fight against global inequities (Hafner and Shiffman, 2013). In view of aging of populations, advantages and disadvantages of geographic location, immigration, and modern socioeconomic dynamics, planning for the future and sustainability of healthcare systems are essential (Tangcharoensathien et al., 2015). Moreover, improving the quality and accessibility of palliative care services can help increase longevity. Systemwide integration of palliative care with extensions of universal health coverage (UHC) will contribute to better management of elderly people (Knaul et al., 2018). In this regard, primary care programs for elderly people and immigrants should be developed within a systemwide approach with consideration of cultural barriers, language, cultural differences, social support, and educational programs (Kwong et al., 2013). The barriers to cultural and economic integration of immigrants and vulnerable groups in the society must be studied (Malmusi, 2015).

Healthcare services must be reorganized to strengthen governance of healthcare. The literature emphasizes that decentralization has improved health equity in developing and developed countries (Sumah et al., 2016). Central coordination and increase in fiscal transfers underlie this improvement. Moreover, an understanding of socioeconomic and organizational contexts aids in the achievement of equity through decentralization (Sumah et al., 2016).

Better coordination and control of health services are essential in the age of technological innovation. However, knowledge, usage, and innovation of healthcare technologies are lacking in developing countries (Kruse et al., 2019). Technological advances will aid in the fight against inequities because geographic dynamics will be considered. Healthcare technologies such as medical artificial intelligence have strong potential in combating poverty in rural and urban parts of developing countries (Wahl et al., 2018). The establishment of multilevel medical artificial intelligence service networks can help improve accessibility of health services in less developed parts of these countries (Guo and Li, 2018). Adaptation of these technologies necessitates strong cooperation among governments, charity organizations, nonprofit organizations, university research institutes, artificial intelligence developers, and medical equipment companies (Guo and Li, 2018).

On the other hand, disease patterns and health conditions in developing countries contribute to considerable inequities in healthcare. Healthcare financing and technology management can help improve accessibility, availability, and utilization of health services. Increasing use of resources outside the medical field in establishing healthcare policy will improve effectiveness and accountability of health policies (Kruk and Freedman, 2008). This chapter provides a close look at equity in different kinds of healthcare-related interventions, financing services, and technologies in developing countries. Equity in healthcare interventions, such as maternal and newborn health, communicable (infectious) diseases, and noncommunicable diseases (NCDs), are examined comparatively. An overview about equity in the distribution of health financing services focuses on the level of out-of-pocket (OOP) and catastrophic health expenditures. Final remarks of this chapter include policy advice to improve healthcare equity in developing countries.

Equity in health interventions in developing countries

The following sections provide a brief overview about health interventions in developing countries that improve healthcare equity. Health interventions that affect every individual and every country should be improved, no matter what type of health system a country may have.

Maternal and newborn health

The state of maternal health is closely related to the accessibility and quality of healthcare services (Koblinsky et al., 2016). Inequities in maternal and newborn health in less developed parts of the world are obvious, in the form of morbidity and mortality rates (Ganle et al., 2014). Thus, maternal health and survival must be improved to improve global health (World Bank, 2019). More than 25% of maternal deaths are attributable to indirect causes. Between the years 2003 and 2009, hemorrhage, hypertensive disorders, and sepsis were responsible for more than half of maternal deaths globally. In other words, maternal mortality in less-developed countries is usually avoidable with health policy interventions (Parata et al., 2009). Inclusive health policies and programs and more funding to reduce maternal mortality at regional and global levels are essential policy interventions to fight against inequities in maternal services (Say et al., 2014).

Current statistics emphasize poor maternal health indicators. The number of maternal deaths per 100,000 live births dropped by 38% globally between the years 2000 and 2017; however, in 2017, the rate of maternal deaths increased in less-developed countries, such as South Sudan, Somalia, Central African Republic, Yemen, Syria, Sudan, Democratic Republic of the Congo, Chad, Afghanistan, Iraq, Haiti, Guinea, Zimbabwe, Nigeria, and Ethiopia (World Health Organization [WHO] Health Topics, 2019). In addition, 94% of all maternal deaths worldwide occur in low- and middle-income countries, and children between the ages of 0 and 14 years in these countries face a high risk of complications from disease. Skilled care before and after childbirth improves maternal and newborn health and saves the lives of women and newborns (de Bernis et al., 2003). However, poor women living in remote and rural areas such as sub-Saharan Africa and South Asia are less likely to receive adequate healthcare, and the numbers of skilled healthcare workers in those areas are low (WHO Health Topics, 2019).

Universal coverage of maternal healthcare services helps reduce inequities in maternal care (Wehrmeister et al., 2016). Figure 3.1 highlights the median coverage of selected health interventions in rural and urban areas of low- and middle-income countries, with regard to satisfaction with family planning, attendance of skilled birth professionals, and antenatal care coverage (at least four visits) between the years 2005 and 2013. Figure 3.1 shows that across low- and middle-income countries, rural areas have lower median coverage than do urban areas for all three indicators. In addition, median coverage is below 80% in rural areas for all indicators.

Less education and lack of skilled birth professionals are the reasons why maternal care is poor in these areas (WHO, 2015). By considering maternal

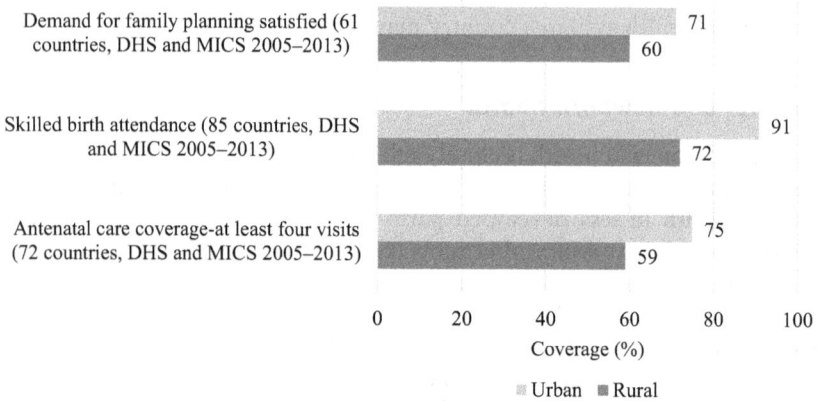

Figure 3.1 Median coverage of selected health interventions, by place of residence, in low- and middle-income countries.

Source: WHO (2015) Tracking universal health coverage. First global monitoring report. WHO and WB. Geneva, Switzerland. Retrieved from: https://apps.who.int/iris/bitstream/handle/10665/174536/9789241564977_eng.pdf;jsessionid=3057C5D4AF2CB5343D9168BE82A37DB8?sequence=1. Accessed on: 3.11.2019. Abbreviations: DHS, Demographic and Health Survey; MICS, Multiple Indicator Cluster Survey.

deaths and geographic differences, maternal healthcare policymakers should provide more focus on rural–urban disparities in developing countries. Of note is that women in less-developed countries have many more pregnancies than do women in developed countries. Thus, their lifetime risk of death from pregnancy-related complications is high (WHO Health Topics, 2019).

Universal access to cesarean section is a key requisite for improving maternal and perinatal outcomes, and inclusive policies are an integral part of the WHO's comprehensive policy for emergency obstetric care (WHO, 2009). The timing and urgency of cesarean section pose major risks. Often, cesarean sections are not performed when needed or are performed when unnecessary. Thus, both over- and underuse of cesarean section can contribute to adverse outcomes (Esteves-Pereira et al., 2016; Ologunde et al., 2014). Maternal deaths and perinatal deaths after cesarean sections are disproportionately high in less-developed countries (Sobhy et al., 2019). In countries with emerging economies – Brazil, Egypt, and Turkey – the rate of cesarean section is reportedly 45%. This high rate necessitates a focus on underlying nonclinical drivers of cesarean sections, such as socioeconomic and psychological reasons (Black and Bhattacharya, 2018).

The number of highly skilled healthcare professionals in developing countries is low, and many developing countries have a shortage of trained doctors. Rural areas are particularly affected negatively by the lack of availability of doctors (Wilson et al., 2011). For these reasons, clinical and nonclinical factors underlying the increase in cesarean delivery rates must be better understood (Zhang et al., 2019). In countries with social and economic underdevelopment, lack of education contributes significantly to the difficulties experienced by women delivering in healthcare facilities (Amutah-Onukagha et al., 2017). In contrast, countries with strong healthcare systems, which provide integrated, continuous, high-quality care, both routinely and in an emergency, are more likely to prevent adverse outcomes faced by women with lower levels of education. In addition to ensuring universal education as a key policy, low-cost, effective interventions implemented within strengthened healthcare systems are needed to prevent maternal morbidity and mortality and to combat maternal inequities (Tunçalp et al., 2014).

Communicable (infectious) diseases

Communicable or infectious diseases are caused by microorganisms such as bacteria, viruses, and parasites that can be spread, directly or indirectly, from one person to another (WHO, 2019a). Wealthy industrialized countries underwent the "epidemiological transition," in which morbidity and mortality resulting from infectious diseases gave way to those resulting from degenerative diseases, but developing countries have not yet achieved that transition (Sanders et al., 2008). Modern sanitation and hygiene practices, effective vaccines, and antibiotics have significantly decreased the burden of such diseases in the developed world; however, infectious diseases remain the most common cause of death globally (Bhutta et al., 2014). Lack of resources to treat and prevent these diseases and the presence of the human immunodeficiency virus (HIV), malaria, and tuberculosis account for the persistent burden of communicable diseases (WHO, 2013). As a result, inequities continue to exist between developed and underdeveloped parts of the world, and better health policymaking is necessary.

Tropical diseases – the infectious diseases that thrive in hot and humid conditions, such as malaria, onchocerciasis, schistosomiasis, and lymphatic filariasis (WHO Health Topics, 2019) – are common problems in poor countries. The economic burden of tropical diseases is high in households and societies because of the high costs of medical care and loss of income (WHO, 2015). Overcoming these diseases would improve economies and development. The establishment of UHC with essential healthcare interventions against tropical diseases, which tend to be overlooked in developed countries, would help achieve global healthcare equity for vulnerable people, as well as for wealthy people; for marginalized people, as well as for privileged people; for the old, as well as for the young; and for women, as well as for men (WHO, 2015).

Figure 3.2 points out existing inequities among developed, developing, and underdeveloped nations by focusing on regional differences, in terms of percentage of coverage for essential services related to communicable

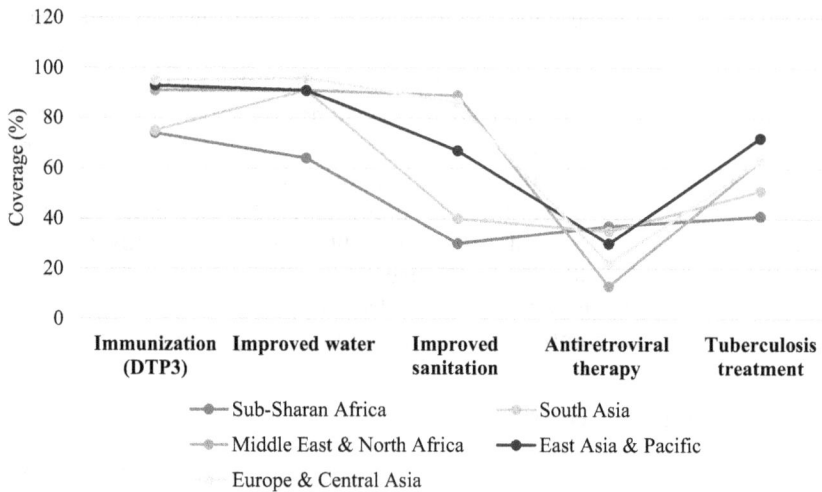

Figure 3.2 Regional coverage in 2013 for essential health services related with communicable diseases.

Source: WHO (2015) Tracking universal health coverage. First global monitoring report. WHO and WB: Switzerland. Geneva. Retrieved from: https://apps.who.int/iris/bitstream/handle/10665/174536/9789241564977_eng.pdf;jsessionid=3057C5D4AF2CB5343D9168BE82A37DB8?sequence=1. Accessed on: 2.10.2019.

(infectious) diseases for the year 2013. Developed European and Central Asian countries have achieved high levels of coverage for immunization (diphtheria–tetanus–pertussis vaccine), improved water and sanitation, and improved tuberculosis treatment. Underdeveloped countries in sub-Saharan Africa and South Asia, in contrast, have low levels of coverage for essential health services.

As a result of emerging and reemerging infections, infectious diseases may spread internationally, and developing countries will face heavy medical and economic burdens (Boutayeb, 2006). The most appropriate strategy to prevent communicable (infectious) diseases and inequities is the development of surveillance networks to detect new patterns of diseases. Further cooperation between government and nongovernment organizations is essential (Sanders et al., 2008). Priority planning with regard to costs of expanding and improving universal coverage of essential healthcare services will be helpful in closing the gap in equity between developed and underdeveloped nations (WHO, 2015).

Noncommunicable diseases

NCDs such as cardiovascular diseases, cancer, and diabetes are affecting millions of people globally. Moreover, it has been reported that more than

75% of deaths from these diseases occur in low- and middle-income countries (Engelgau et al., 2018). Many underdeveloped countries are also burdened with communicable diseases such as HIV/acquired immunodeficiency syndrome, malaria, and tuberculosis. NCDs are a drain on government budgets and increase poverty and inequities in developing countries (WHO, 2019b).

According to the Global Burden of Diseases study for the year 2013, the prevalence of NCDs has increased, and high body mass index is the leading risk factor for NCDs in women in nearly all countries in the Americas, North Africa, and the Middle East. Moreover, for men, high systolic blood pressure and tobacco use are the leading risks for NCDs in nearly all high-income countries and in North Africa, the Middle East, Europe, and Asia (Global Burden of Disease, 2013).

The current status of and future predictions about NCDs are alarming, especially for developing countries. Figure 3.3 indicates that increasing trend of NCDs will continue and that 25 million people will be affected by NCDs in the developing world in the year 2020.

Diabetes is one of the leading NCDs. Sedentary lifestyles, obesity, and aging of the population contribute to the increase in the prevalence of diabetes (Katon, 2008). Figure 3.4 indicates diabetes prevalence for the years 2000 and 2030 in different countries, including developing nations. Predictions about diabetes prevalence in developing countries are of considerable interest; in particular, the prevalence is expected to increase in India and China by 2030. These countries are also pharmerging nations, and expenditures for healthcare and pharmaceuticals are growing fast. It is obvious that the prevalence of diabetes has increased since 2000 and

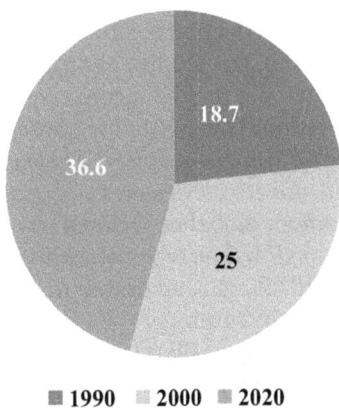

■ 1990   ▨ 2000   ■ 2020

Figure 3.3 Noncommunicable diseases in developing countries (in millions).

Source: World Health Organization (2003). Diet, Nutrition and the prevention of Chronic Diseases. In Technical report Series 916 Geneva, World Health Organization, 2003.

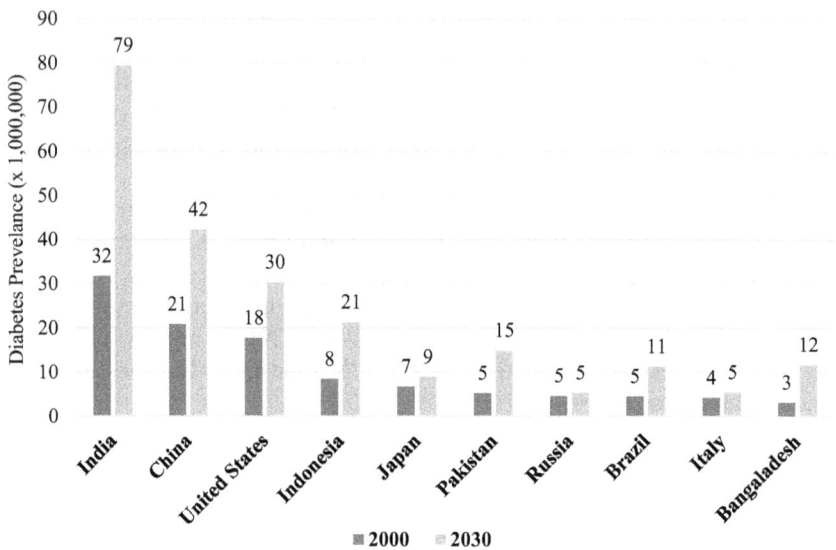

Figure 3.4 Diabetes prevalence (× 10⁶).

Source: International Diabetes Federation (IDF): Action Now: A joint initiative WHO and IDF. Retrieved from: www.idf.org. Accessed on: 16.8.2019.

is expected to continue rising through 2030 in most developing countries (IDF, 2019).

Treatment of NCDs is costly, and these diseases have social and economic consequences that affect individuals, households, and society as a whole. They exacerbate healthcare inequity between and within countries (Boutayeb and Boutayeb, 2005). Inclusive and effective healthcare policies are essential in handling the high burden of NCDs. Studies about tackling socioeconomic inequalities and NCDs in low- and middle-income countries have shown that better economic and educational outcomes for households reduce inequities in health. However, lack of treatment for NCDs leads to reduced income levels of households and poverty (Niessen et al., 2018). Despite the increase in NCDs, knowledge about global or regional coverage of NCDs, such as diabetes, is sparse, and no global or regional estimates of diabetes treatment coverage exist (WHO, 2015). It is advisable to include treatment for diabetes and other costly NCDs in coverage.

Programs related to UHC of NCDs should especially target susceptible populations, which include elderly people and people with risk factors for NCDs (Niessen et al., 2018). Many prevention and primary care policies have options with which to modify key risks (Global Burden of Disease, 2018). NCDs such as diabetes boost multimorbidity of cardiovascular diseases and cancer; thus, healthcare policymakers should pay particular attention to the association between equity and multimorbidity of NCDs. Cost-effective strategies are necessary for early diagnosis and promotion of a healthy diet, physical activity, and no alcohol (Boutayeb et al., 2013). Successful lessons learned from other countries, such as tobacco control in Turkey, are critical for other developing countries. Turkey's successful experience with tobacco control shows that the strong link between the global and national network is essential in minimizing causes of NCDs. Turkey's effective tobacco control policies, with strong leadership and strong collaborations between healthcare professionals, policymakers, and pharmaceutical companies, can serve as a role model for other developing countries (Hoe et al., 2019).

New technologies will be helpful in overcoming regional disparities in the struggle to manage the increasing burden of NCDs. Mobile health technologies are a promising tool to address access, coverage, and equity gaps in developing countries and low-resource settings (Sondaal et al., 2016). They are useful in combating NCDs in underdeveloped countries. However, more effort is necessary for effective usage of these technologies to improve health in developing countries, especially in rural areas (Beratarrechea et al., 2014). All-in-all, expanded quality service coverage, public education programs, and recent technology advances to help raise awareness of the signs and symptoms of NCDs (Cowie et al., 2014) are policy options to improve efficiency, equity, coverage, and quality of health services. A special focus on cardiovascular disease, cancer, chronic respiratory disease, diabetes, and their risk factors is necessary to fight against healthcare inequities in developing countries (WHO, 2013).

Equity in distribution of health financing in developing countries

Developing countries are faced with financial hardships because of the aging of their populations and changes in disease patterns from communicable diseases to noncommunicable ones (Mohan et al., 2019). These epidemiological changes and disease burdens will have economic effects on the social security systems (Arredondo and Aviles, 2015). Thus, inclusive financing policies and financial resource allocation are critical strategies in the health policymaking process. Moreover, according to projections about future global health spending, healthcare expenses will increase and must be monitored. Global healthcare spending is projected to increase from US$10 trillion in 2015 to US$20 trillion in 2040. Per capita healthcare spending was projected to rise fastest in upper-middle-income countries, at an average of 4.2% (estimated range, 3.4%–5.1%) per year, followed by lower-middle-income countries and low-income countries. According to alternative scenarios, UHC will be applied to between 5.1 billion people (estimated range, 4.9–5.3 billion people) and 5.6 billion people (estimated range, 5.3–5.8 billion people) in 2030 (Global Burden of Disease, 2018). With high healthcare expenditures, financial protection of families and inclusive health financing policies must be the core considerations of healthcare system evaluations (Quintal, 2019).

UHC is defined as the provision of high-quality and needed health services without financial hardship. Successful prepayment helps protect households from financial and economic strains (WHO, 2010). OOP healthcare payment is defined as direct payment made to healthcare providers by patients at the time they receive healthcare services. These payments may be in the form of taxes, insurance premiums, or contributions (Xu et al., 2003). Increases in OOP payments have a number of disadvantages; among them is that the expenses discourage poor people from seeking care. Thus, the increases in OOP expenses and the differences in OOP expenditures between rich and poor populations provide many insights about health financing equity (WHO, 2014).

The design of UHC is at the core of efforts to strengthen equity in healthcare. In developing countries, equity can be achieved by improvements in the health status of people and in the distribution of healthcare services (WHO, 2015). In UHC, all people receive the healthcare services they need, including health initiatives to improve population health, such as antitobacco policies, illness prevention, and the provision of treatment, rehabilitation, and palliative care (WHO, 2010; 2015).

Quality of care, provision of essential health services, and financial coverage are elements of UHC (WHO, 2010). These three dimensions are typically represented in what has come to be known as the "coverage cube" (Figure 3.5). In many countries, filling the cube is a struggle: for example, it is difficult to keep a level of coverage despite rising costs. Thus, UHC is a journey in itself, not a destination (WHO, 2015). Dynamic and continuous improvement in UHC must be consistent with demographic, epidemiological, and technological changes worldwide (Savedoff et al., 2012). In each dimensions of this cube, policymakers need to base decisions on fairness and equity. When expanding priority services, policymakers must decide which services to include. When covering more people, decisionmakers must make a critical preference about whom to cover first. When reducing OOP expenses, policymakers must choose between different prepayment mechanisms. Every country has its own demographic, epidemiological, and technological dynamics, and no single form of UHC is suitable for every country (WHO, 2014).

Catastrophic expenditure and impoverishment expenditure

Healthcare expenditure is catastrophic when a household must reduce its expenditures on basic necessities to accommodate increasing healthcare costs (Xu et al., 2003). However, there is no internationally consensus about the acceptable threshold of household healthcare expenditures. Some researchers considered 5%–20% of total household income as the threshold.

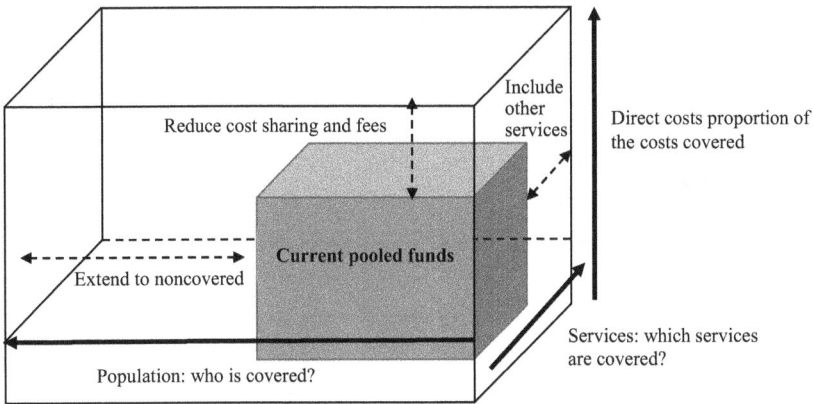

Figure 3.5 Three dimensions to consider when moving toward UHC.

Source: WHO (2010). The World Health Report 2010. Health systems financing: the path to universal coverage. World Health Organization: Geneva, 2010.

Others consider the threshold to be 40% of total household income. Rising OOP expenditures contribute to the impoverishment of households (Xu et al., 2003). Global monitoring of financial protection against catastrophic and impoverishment effects of OOP expenditures is critical because measurement methods differ and the threshold has not been established (Hsu et al., 2018). The distribution of OOP expenditures and their catastrophic effects in 146 countries from all World Bank--defined income groups demonstrate that OOP expenditures tend to rise among poor people and that catastrophic expenditures tend to be concentrated among poor people in relation to income. Among wealthy people, in contrast, catastrophic OOP expenditures tend to be concentrated in relation to consumption. OOP expenditures cause high levels of impoverishment among low-income countries (Wagstaff et al., 2019). Healthcare policymakers should consider income and other local characteristics while planning healthcare services because financial resource constraints and inequities between rural and urban areas are obvious in underdeveloped countries (Strasser et al., 2016).

Figure 3.6 depicts median per capita OOP expenditures on health, in 2011 international dollars, in different geographic regions. Wealthy countries tend to have more OOP expenses than do poorer ones. High-income populations from countries in North America, East Asia, and the Pacific region are faced with high OOP expenditures. Upper-middle-income countries, which include developing nations, are at risk for high OOP spending; this is especially true for countries in the Middle East and North Africa.

Continuous monitoring of the level of UHC and its impoverishing effects on households, as well as monitoring of the health status and health expenditures of households, is one of the ways to enhance equities in health

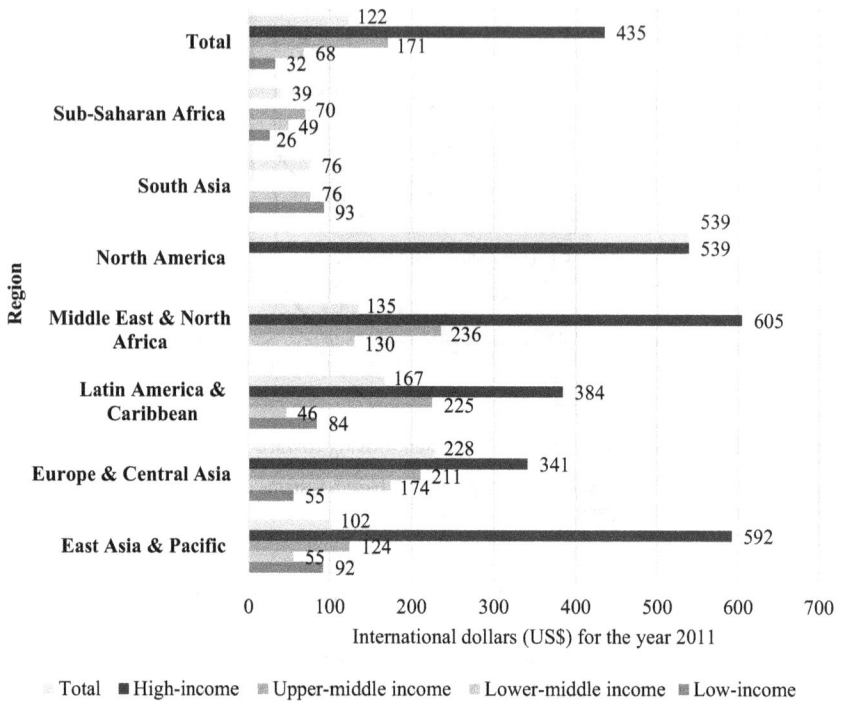

Figure 3.6 Median per capita OOP expenditures on health, 2011 international dollars, latest year.

Source: Wagstaff A, Eozenou P, Smitz M. (2019) Out-of-Pocket Expenditures on Health: A Global Stocktake Policy Research Working Papers. No. 8808.

services distribution (Hosseinpoor and Bergen, 2019). In a joint study of 2014, the WHO and the World Bank monitored progress toward UHC by focusing on middle-income countries; the findings highlight the current status of UHC (WHO and World Bank, 2014). In this study, catastrophic expenditure is defined as OOP expenditures equal to or exceeding 25% of total household expenditure. Figure 3.7 shows that catastrophic expenditure tends to be higher among the quantiles in which spending on healthcare services is high. The median catastrophic expenditure is 1% in the lowest spending quantile and 2.7% in the highest spending quantile.

The level of healthcare expenditures changes according to the type of healthcare service. Healthcare expenditures are highest for in- and outpatient services and for medicines (Stenberg et al., 2018). High costs of research and development, driven by the pharmaceutical sector, increase in the consumption of healthcare services (Xiong et al., 2019). Pharmaceutical expenditures constitute the highest among of OOP expenditures. In their 2018 global health financing report, Xu et al. (2018) stated inpatient care, outpatient

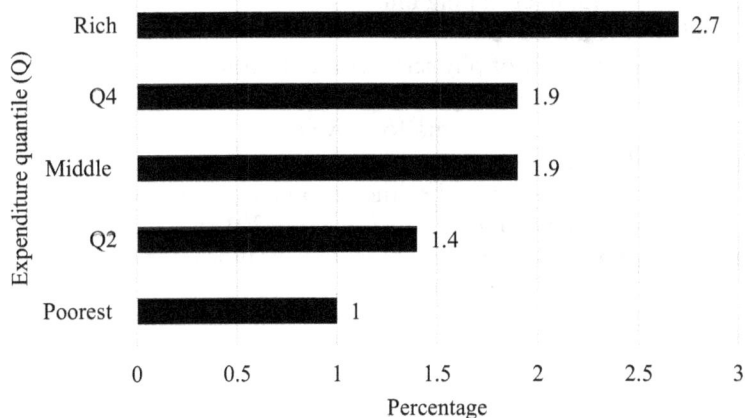

Figure 3.7 Catastrophic health spending by expenditure quantile (Q), mean values of selected 37 low- and middle-income countries (headcount ratio, percentage).

Source: World Health Organization and World Bank Group (2014). Monitoring progress toward universal health coverage at country and global levels. Framework measures and targets. Geneva: World Health Organization and International Bank for Reconstruction and Development/ World Bank, 2014.

care, and medicines and medical supplies together account for more than 70% of healthcare spending (Xu et al., 2018). Affordability and access to medicines are limited particularly in countries where a significant portion of pharmaceutical spending is OOP. Changes in pharmaceutical pricing increase the need for continuous monitoring by healthcare policymakers, and affordability and accessibility to medicines must be considered by pharmaceutical policymakers (Hasan et al., 2019). Transparency and accountability in national pharmaceutical markets will improve access to medicines, and safe, effective, good-quality medicines will improve population health. Of note also is that high levels of transparency and accountability are critical for minimizing fraud in the pharmaceutical sector (Paschke et al., 2018). Thus, fraud detection must be incorporated into the pharmaceutical market design process.

Pharmaceutical development is dynamic and is advancing rapidly. Collaborative decision-making in this multifaceted sector will promote awareness of current trends and new technologies (Nematollahi et al., 2017). The contributions of physicians, other healthcare providers, and professionals in related fields to the pharmaceutical market design processes increase interactions between decisionmakers. Such an integrated decision-making process will enable policymakers to understand consumer needs and to better handle inequities (Sendyona et al., 2016). In developing countries, pharmacists play a leading role in healthcare, providing multiple services in patient care that enhance health outcomes and reduce healthcare costs.

Their guidance is helpful in curtailing unnecessary prescribing and usage of antibiotics (Sakeena et al., 2018).

In addition to involvement of physicians, other healthcare providers, and professionals in related fields in pharmaceutical design process, rational policymaking will create cost benefits for developing countries (Walt and Gilson, 1994). Health technology assessment, commonly used in developed countries, are essential aspects of healthcare policymaking and must be implemented in developing countries (Awaisu et al., 2018). Rational policy-making in the pharmaceutical market will reduce healthcare inequities and enable effective usage of limited financial resources in developing countries (Hu and Mossialos, 2016). The following section includes specific policy suggestions for improving equity in developing countries.

Policy advice to improve equities in developing countries

Every country has its own healthcare dynamics and healthcare regulations. Good health and well-being are fundamental for the prosperity of nations (Tavares, 2017). In all countries, citizens' access to healthcare services and medicines depends on their public healthcare system and the global pharmaceutical market (Pezzola and Sweet, 2016). It is estimated that at least 400 million people are lacking essential healthcare services, such as family planning and immunization. Moreover, catastrophic healthcare expenditures are common among people who use healthcare services (WHO, 2015). Developing countries must assess the accessibility of medicines in healthcare regulations (Pezzola and Sweet, 2016).

There has been a growing interest in UHC, in as much as quality health services are lacking and financial coverage is inadequate for high proportions of populations in low- and middle-income countries (WHO, 2015). Three objectives of UHC must be achieved to improve equity in healthcare in each country: increasing the population that is covered by pooled funds, increasing the proportion of direct healthcare costs covered by pooled funds, and increasing the number of healthcare services covered by those funds (WHO, 2010).

OOP expenditures would be distributed fairly in an egalitarian society (O'Donnell et al., 2008; Wagstaff et al., 1989). UHC is desirable in all coun-tries, but because of global changes in sociodemographic, economic, and technological trends, UHC is also necessary to combat inequities in health and distribution of financial resources (Reich et al., 2016). UHC is a long-term policy engagement for which both technological knowledge and polit-ical know-how are needed. Technical solutions to deal with inequities must be developed in pragmatic and innovative policymaking that accounts for national economies and social expectations (Reich et al., 2016).

Today, the world's center of economic gravity is changing. Developing and emerging economies are key drivers of global economic growth. Moreover, the nature of development financing is changing, and developing countries are becoming important components of international trade and finance (Slesman et al., 2019). In addition to economic dynamics, population dynamics, such as migration flow, necessitates strong commitment to improve equity in developing countries. The current flow of immigrants into developing countries causes populations to become ethnically diverse and increases health inequalities. Proactive leadership and inclusive actions with increasing global collaborations will improve immigrants' access to healthcare services (Ledoux et al., 2018)

The transformational leadership of government organizations in different fields of public services should provide continuity and promote health equity. Developing countries have both growing economies and growing populations. Social, political, and economic trends affect decision-making processes in all fields, including decisions involving equal distribution of health resources (Xu et al., 2018). Most developing countries are still in the process of industrialization, and welfare programs need to mature. Thus, healthcare policymaking processes are strongly affected by politically motivated strategies rather than by need to reduce inequities in society (Bugra, 2018). Advisable policies for tackling health inequities include equity-oriented economic growth and labor market policies, tax credits for low-income families, minimum salary levels to guarantee a living wage, reduction in gender-specific income differences, promotion of women's employment, expansion of child care and preschool care, provision of equal education opportunities for adults, improvement in health literacy, fair regulations in pensions that enable older adults to achieve necessary health services, and strong primary care systems (Dahlgren et al., 2006).

Continuous monitoring of UHC is an implicit part of assessing the performance of a healthcare system. Tracking trends and inequalities in the healthcare system, coverage, risk factors, and health outcomes is essential (Reich et al., 2016; Dahlgren et al., 2006). Regional and geographic disparities in developing countries must be assessed to determine usage and financing of healthcare services. Overcoming geographic barriers to high-quality healthcare services must be an integral part of the policymaking process (de Souza et al., 2016). The distributional effects of public and private financing on healthcare services, daycare, school lunches, services for older adults, and other essential welfare services must be evaluated. Continuous equity follow-up is necessary in every country (Hosseinpoor et al., 2015).

Today, there is an increasing recognition reducing poverty in high- and middle-income countries has less to do with economic resources and more to do with political actors, the degree of political solidarity, and trust in the society (Dhalgren et al., 2006). The level of democratization of a country plays a vital role in equal distribution of healthcare resources and expenditures in the community. Promoting democracy improves health outcomes (Okada, 2018). Healthcare policymakers determine policies by considering expectations of their supporters in less democratized countries. In countries with populist governments, policymaking processes continue to produce inequities in healthcare systems (Eckermann, 2017). The weakness of democratic institutions hampers the monitoring and detection of healthcare inequities and indicates to populist politicians that future policies should be determined according to the preferences of median voters (Acemoglu et al., 2013). Populist politicians' priorities with regard to healthcare policies are to satisfy their supporters and increase the visibility of their policies (Agartan and Kuhlmann, 2019). Establishment of transparent, accountable, and independent healthcare policymaking and social security system is necessary for equal distribution of resources in healthcare.

The pharmaceutical market is a costly area of healthcare services. To solve the problems in healthcare financing in developing countries, a more thorough understanding of inequities in the pharmaceutical market is essential (Greene, 2011). Tight market control strategies are obviously necessary because the pharmaceutical market is highly competitive and has fascinating growth potential in emerging economies. In addition, developing countries are exciting contexts for the pharmaceutical market (Gereffi, 2017). The absence of a developmental commitment to a pharmaceutical sector--specific policy is a problem in developing countries (Dorlach, 2016). Extending the growth potential of the generic drug market and incorporating equity principles into pharmaceutical marketing plans and policymaking processes will enable equal distribution of resources. Of note is that the increasing level of pharmaceutical spending has a negative effect on gross domestic product per capita, especially in the countries with limited economic freedom (Kumru and Top, 2018). Improvements in the level of democracy and transparency are strongly advisable for dealing with high costs and for ensuring equity in the pharmaceutical market. Moreover, increases in knowledge and big data provide metrics suitable for monitoring key performance indicators in the pharmaceutical market (Seebode et al., 2013). With the use of new technologies and big data, it is possible to analyze the number of adverse drug reactions and a population's response to adverse drug reactions. This will be beneficial in establishing medicine-based companion diagnostics services (Auffray et al., 2016).

The most important recommendation is to discuss what additional steps are necessary to create an environment in which healthcare services are accessible to all people. Ensuring availability and accessibility of healthcare services while considering costs is the only way of promoting equity in the distribution of healthcare services. Experiences in healthcare reform learned from pharmerging countries are of considerable interest to equity researchers. The following chapter provides a deep understanding of equity experiences learned from developing countries in view of health reform.

References

Acemoglu D, Egorov G, Sonin K. (2013) A political theory of populism. *Quarterly Journal of Economics* 128(2):771–805.

Agartan TI, Kuhlmann E. (2019) New public management, physicians and populism: Turkey's experience with health reforms. *Sociology of Health & Illness* 41(7):1410–1425.

Amutah-Onukagha N, Rodriguez M, Opara I, Gardner M, Assan MA, Hammond R, Plata J, Pierre K, Farag E. (2017) Progresses and challenges of utilizing traditional birth attendants in maternal and child health in Nigeria. *International Journal of MCH and AIDS* 6(2):130–138.

Arredondo A, Aviles R. (2015) Costs and epidemiological changes of chronic diseases: Implications and challenges for health systems. *PLoS ONE* 10(3):e0118611.

Auffray C, Balling R, Barroso I, Bencze L, Benson M, Bergeron J. et al. (2016) Making sense of big data in health research: Towards an EU action plan. *Genome Medicine* 8(71):1–13.

Awaisu A. Niewada M, Greenberg D. (2018) Drug policy research and health technology assessment in Central and Eastern Europe, Western Asia, and Africa: The interface between research evidence, policy, and practice. *Value in Health Regional Issues* 16:119–120.

Beratarrechea A, Lee AG, Willner JM, Jahangir E, Ciapponi A, Rubinstein A. (2014) The impact of mobile health interventions on chronic disease outcomes in developing countries: A systematic review. *Telemedicine and e-Health* 20(1):75–82.

Bhutta ZA, Sommerfeld J, Lassi ZS, Salam RA, Das JK. (2014) Global burden, distribution, and interventions for infectious diseases of poverty. *Infectious Diseases of Poverty* 3(21):1–7.

Black M, Bhattacharya S. (2018) Cesarean section in China, Taiwan, and Hong Kong—A safe choice for women and clinicians? *PLoS Medicine* 15(10):e1002676.

Boutayeb A, Boutayeb S, Boutayeb W. (2013) Multi-morbidity of non-communicable diseases and equity in WHO Eastern Mediterranean countries. *International Journal for Equity in Health* 12(60):1–13.

Boutayeb A, Boutayeb S. (2005) The burden of non-communicable diseases in developing countries. *International Journal for Equity in Health* 4(1):1–8.

Boutayeb A. (2006) The double burden of communicable and non-communicable diseases in developing countries. *Transactions of the Royal Society of Tropical Medicine and Hygiene* 100(3):191–199.

Bugra A. (2018) Social policy and different dimensions of inequality in Turkey: A historical overview. *Journal of Balkan and Near Eastern Studies* 20(4):318–331.

Cowie MR, Anker SD, Cleland JGF, Michael Felker G, Filippatos G, Jaarsma T, Jourdain P, Knight E, Massie B, Ponikowski P, López-Sendón J. (2014) Improving care for patients with acute heart failure: Before, during and after hospitalization. *ESC Heart Failure* 1(2):110–145.

Dahlgren G, Whitehead M. WHO Collaborating Centre for Policy Research on Social Determinants of Health University of Liverpool, et al. (2006) European strategies for tackling social inequities in health: Levelling up Part 2. World Health Organization Regional Office for Europe, Copenhagen, Denmark.

de Bernis L, Sherratt DR, AbouZahr C, van Lerberghe WV. (2003) Skilled attendants for pregnancy, childbirth and postnatal care. *British Medical Bulletin* 67(1):39–57.

de Souza JA, Hunt B, Asirwa FC, Adebamowo C, Lopes G. (2016) Global health equity: Cancer care outcome disparities in high-, middle-, and low-income countries. *Journal of Clinical Oncology* 34(1):6–13.

Dorlach T. (2016) The AKP between populism and neoliberalism: Lessons from pharmaceutical policy. *New Perspectives on Turkey* 55:55–83.

Eckermann E. (2017) Global health promotion in the era of "galloping populism" *Health Promotion International* 32(3):415–418.

Engelgau MM, Rosenthal JP, Newsome BJ, Price LS, Belis D, Mensah GA. (2018) Noncommunicable Diseases in low- and middle-income countries: A strategic approach to develop a global implementation research workforce. *Global Health* 13(2):131–137.

Esteves-Pereira AP, Deneux-Tharaux C, Nakamura-Pereira M, Saucedo M, Bouvier-Colle MH, et al. (2016) Caesarean delivery and postpartum maternal mortality: A population-based case control study in Brazil. *PLoS One* 11(4):e0153396.

Ganle JK, Parker M, Fitzpatrick R, Otupiri E. (2014) Inequities in accessibility to and utilisation of maternal health services in Ghana after user-fee exemption: A descriptive study. *International Journal for Equity in Health* 13(89):1–19.

Gereffi G. (2017) *The pharmaceutical industry and dependency in the third world. Princeton Legacy Library*. Princeton University Press: Princeton, New Jersey, USA.

Global Burden of Disease (GBD). (2013) Risk Factors Collaborators (2015). Global, regional, and national comparative risk assessment of 79 behavioral, environmental and occupational, and metabolic risks or clusters of risks in 188 countries, 1990–2013: A systematic analysis for the Global Burden of Disease Study 2013. *The Lancet* 386(10010):2287–2323.

Global Burden of Disease (GBD). (2018) Health Financing Collaborator Network (2018) Trends in future health financing and coverage: Future health spending and universal health coverage in 188 countries, 2016–40. *The Lancet* 361(10132):1783–1798.

Greene JA. (2011) Making medicines essential: The emergent centrality of pharmaceuticals in global health. *BioSocieties* 6(1):10–33.

Guo J, Li B. (2018) The application of medical artificial intelligence technology in rural areas of developing countries. *Health Equity* 2(1):174–181.

Hafner T, Shiffman J. (2013) The emergence of global attention to health systems strengthening. *Health Policy and Planning* 28(1):41–50.

Hasan SS, Kow CS, Dawoud D, Mohamed O, Baines D, Babar ZUD (2019). Pharmaceutical policy reforms to regulate drug prices in the Asia Pacific Region: The case of Australia, China, India, Malaysia, New Zealand, and South Korea. *Value in Health Regional Issues* 18:18–23.

Hoe C, Rodriguez DC, Uzumcuoglu Y, Hyder AA. (2019) Understanding political priority development for public health issues in Turkey: Lessons from tobacco control and road safety. *Health Research Policy and Systems* 17(13):1–13.

Hosseinpoor A.R., Bergen N. (2019) Health inequality monitoring: A practical application of population health monitoring. In: Verschuuren M., van Oers H. (eds) *Population Health Monitoring*. Springer: Cham.

Hosseinpoor AR, Bergen N, Schlotheuber A. (2015) Promoting health equity: WHO health inequality monitoring at global and national levels. *Global Health Action* 8(1):1–8.

Hsu J. Flores G, Evans D, Mills A, Hanson K. (2018) Measuring financial protection against catastrophic health expenditures: Methodological challenges for global monitoring. *International Journal for Equity in Health* 17(69):1–13.

Hu J, Mossialos E. (2016) Pharmaceutical pricing and reimbursement in China: When the whole is less than the sum of its parts. *Health Policy* 120(5):519–534.

International Diabetes Federation (IDF): Action Now: A Joint Initiative WHO and IDF. Retrieved from: www.idf.org. Accessed on: 16.8.2019.

Katon WJ. (2008) The comorbidity of diabetes mellitus and depression. *The American Journal of Medicine* 121(11):S8–S15.

Knaul FM, Farmer PE, Krakauer EL, De Lima L, Bhadelia A. et al. (2018) Alleviating the access abyss in palliative care and pain relief—An imperative of universal health coverage. *The Lancet* 391(10128):1391–1454.

Koblinsky M, Moyer CA, Calvert C, Campbell J (2016) Quality maternity care for every woman, everywhere: A call to action. *The Lancet* 388(10057):5–11.

Kruk ME, Freedman LP. (2008) Assessing health system performance in developing countries: A review of the literature. *Health Policy* 85(3):263–276.

Kruse C, Betancourt J, Ortiz S, Luna SMV (2019) Barriers to the use of mobile health in improving health outcomes in developing countries: Systematic review. *Journal of Medical Internet Research* 21(10):e13263.

Kumru S, Top M. (2018) Pricing and reimbursement of generic pharmaceuticals in Turkey: Evaluation of hypertension drugs from 2007 to 2013. *Health Policy and Technology* 7(2):182–193.

Kwong K, Chung H, Cheal K, Chou JC, Chen T. (2013) Depression care management for Chinese Americans in primary care: A feasibility pilot study. *Community Mental Health Journal* 49(2):157–165.

Ledoux C, Pilot E, Diaz E, Krafft T. (2018) Migrants' access to healthcare services within the European Union: A content analysis of policy documents in Ireland, Portugal and Spain. *Globalization and Health* 14(57):1–11.

Lee A, Kiyu A, Milman HM, Jimenez J. (2007) Improving health and building human capital through an effective primary care system. *Journal of Urban Health* 84:75–85.

Malmusi D. (2015) Immigrants' health and health inequality by type of integration policies in European countries. *European Journal of Public Health* 25(2):293–299.

Mitsumori Y. (2019) Growth factors and prospects of two "pharmerging" countries: A comparative study of the pharmaceutical industries of India and Bangladesh, 2019 8th International Congress on Advanced Applied Informatics (IIAI-AAI), Toyama, Japan, 2019, pp. 756–761. doi: 10.1109/IIAI-AAI.2019.00155.

Mohan P, Mohan SB, Dutta M. (2019) Communicable or noncommunicable diseases? Building strong primary health care systems to address double burden of disease in India. *Journal of Family Medicine and Primary Care* 8(2):326–329.

Nematollahi MR, Hosseini-Motlagh SM, Heydari J. (2017) Economic and social collaborative decision-making on visit interval and service level in a two-echelon pharmaceutical supply chain. *Journal of Cleaner Production* 142(4):3956–3969.

Niessen LW, Mohan D, Akuoku JK, Mirelman AJ, Ahmed S, Koehlmoos TP, Trujillo A, Khan J, Peters DH. (2018) Tackling socioeconomic inequalities and non-communicable diseases in low-income and middle-income countries under the Sustainable Development agenda. *The Lancet* 391(10134):2036–2046.

O'Donnell O, van Doorslaer E, Wagstaff A, Lindelow M. (2008) *Analyzing health equity using household survey data. A guide to techniques and their implementation.* The World Bank. Washington, D.C.

Okada K. (2018) Health and political regimes: Evidence from quantile regression. *Economic Systems* 42(2):307–319.

Ologunde R, Vogel JP, Cherian MN, Sbaiti M, Merialdi M, Yeats J. (2014) Assessment of cesarean delivery availability in 26 low- and middle-income countries: A cross-sectional study. *American Journal of Obstetrics and Gynecology* 211(5):e1–12.

Parata N, Graff M, Graves A, Potts M. (2009) Avoidable maternal deaths: Three ways to help now. *Global Public Health* 4(6):575–587.

Paschke A, Dimancesco D, Vian T, Kohler JC, Forte G. (2018) Increasing transparency and accountability in national pharmaceutical systems. *Bulletin of the World Health Organization* 96(11):782–791.

Pezzola A, Sweet CM. (2016) Global pharmaceutical regulation: The challenge of integration for developing states. *Globalization and Health* 12(85):1–18.

Quintal C. (2019) Evaluation of catastrophic health expenditure in a high-income country: Incidence versus inequalities. *International Journal for Equity in Health* 18(145):1–11.

Reich MR, Harris J, Ikegami N, Maeda A, Cashin C, Araujo EC, Takemi K, Evans TG. (2016) Moving towards universal health coverage: Lessons from 11 country studies. *The Lancet* 387(10020):811–816.

Sakeena MHF, Bennett AA, McLachlan AJ. (2018). Enhancing pharmacists' role in developing countries to overcome the challenge of antimicrobial resistance: A narrative review. *Antimicrobial Resistance & Infection Control* 7(63):1–11.

Sanders JW, Fuhrer GS, Johnson MD, Riddle MS. (2008) The epidemiological transition: The current status of infectious diseases in the developed world versus the developing world. *Science Progress* 91(1):1–37.

Savedoff WD, de Ferranti D, Smith AL, Fan V. (2012). Political and economic aspects of the transition to universal health coverage. *The Lancet* 380(9845):924–932.

Say L, Chou D, Gemmill A, Tunçalp Ö, Moller AB, Daniels J, Gülmezoglu AM, Temmerman M, Alkema L. (2014) Global causes of maternal death: A WHO systematic analysis. *The Lancet Global Health* 2(6):e323–e333.

Schmitt M, Blue A, Aschenbrener CA, Viggiano TR. (2011) Core competencies for interprofessional collaborative practice: Reforming health care by transforming health professionals' education. *Academic Medicine* 86(11):1351. https://doi.org/10.1097/ACM.0b013e3182308e39.

Seebode C, Ort M, Regenbrecht C, Peuker M. (2013) BIG DATA infrastructures for pharmaceutical research. IEEE International Conference on Big Data. doi: 10.1109/BigData.2013.6691759.

Sendyona S, Odeyemi I, Maman K. (2016) Perceptions and factors affecting pharmaceutical market access: Results from a literature review and survey of stakeholders in different settings. *Journal of Market Access & Health Policy* 4(1):1–10.

Sitthi-Amorn C, Somrongthong R. (2000) Strengthening health research capacity in developing countries: A critical element for achieving health equity. *British Medical Journal* 321(7264):813–817.

Slesman L, Baharumshah AZ, Azman-Saini WNW. (2019) Political institutions and finance-growth nexus in emerging markets and developing countries: A tale of one threshold. *The Quarterly Review of Economics and Finance* 72:80–100.

Sobhy S, Arroyo-Manzano D, Murugesu N, Karthikeyan G, Kumar V, Kaur I, Fernandez E, Gundabattula SR, Betran AP, Khan K, Zamora J, Thangaratinam S. (2019) Maternal and perinatal mortality and complications associated with cae-sarean section in low-income and middle-income countries: A systematic review and meta-analysis. *The Lancet* 393(10184):1973–1982.

Sondaal SFV, Browne JL, Amoakoh-Coleman M, Borgstein A, Miltenburg AS, Verwijs M, Klipstein-Grobusch K. (2016) Assessing the effect of mHealth interventions in improving maternal and neonatal care in low- and middle-income countries: A systematic review. *PLoS One* 11(5): e0154664.

Stenberg K, Lauer JA, Gkountouras G, Fitzpatrick C, Stanciole A. (2018) Econometric estimation of WHO-CHOICE country-specific costs for inpatient and outpatient health service delivery. *Cost Effectiveness and Resource Allocation* 16(11):1–15.

Strasser R, Kam SM, Regalado SM. (2016) Rural health care access and policy in developing countries. *Annual Review of Public Health* 37:395–412.

Sumah AH, Baatiema L, Abimbola S. (2016) The impacts of decentralisation on health-related equity: A systematic review of the evidence. *Health Policy* 120(10):1183–1192.

Tangcharoensathien V, Mills A, Palu T. (2015) Accelerating health equity: The key role of universal health coverage in the Sustainable Development Goals. *BMC Medicine* 13(101):1–5.

Tavares AI. (2017). Infant mortality in Europe, socio-economic determinants based on aggregate data. *Applied Economics Letters* 24(21):1588–1596.

Tunçalp Ö, Souza JP, Hindin MJ, Santos CA, Oliveira TH, Vogel JP, Togoobaatar G, Ha DQ, Say L, Gülmezoglu AM. On behalf of the WHO multicountry survey on maternal and newborn health research network. (2014) Education and severe maternal outcomes in developing countries: A multicountry cross-sectional survey. *British Journal of Obstetrics and Gynaecology* 121(1):57–65.

Wagstaff A, Eozenou P, Smitz M. (2019) Out-of-Pocket Expenditures on Health: A Global Stocktake. Policy Research Working Papers. No. 8808.

Wagstaff A, van Doorslaer E, Paci P. (1989) Equity in the finance and delivery of health care: Some tentative cross-country comparisons. *Oxford Review of Economic Policy* 5(1):89–112.

Wahl B, Cossy-Gantner A, Germann S, Schwalbe NR. (2018) Artificial intelligence (AI) and global health: How can AI contribute to health in resource-poor settings? *BMJ Global Health* 3(4):e000798. doi:10.1136/bmjgh-2018-000798.

Walt G, Gilson L. (1994) Reforming the health sector in developing countries: The central role of policy analysis. *Health Policy and Planning* 9(4):353–370.

Wehrmeister FC, Restrepo-Mendez MC, Franca GVA, Victora CG, Barros AJD. (2016) Summary indices for monitoring universal coverage in maternal and child health care. *Bulletin of the World Health Organization* 94(12): 903–912.

Wilson A, Lissauer D, Thangaratinam S, Khan KS, MacArthur C, Coomarasamy A. (2011) A comparison of clinical officers with medical doctors on outcomes of caesarean section in the developing world: Meta-analysis of controlled studies. *British Medical Journal* 342:d2600.

World Bank (WB) (2019) Trends in maternal mortality 2000 to 2017: Estimates by WHO, UNICEF, UNFPA, World Bank Group and the United Nations Population Division (Vol. 2) (English). Washington, D.C.: World Bank Group. http://documents. worldbank.org/curated/en/793971568908763231/Trends-in-maternal-mortality-2000-to-2017-Estimates-by-WHO-UNICEF-UNFPA-World-Bank-Group-and-the-United-Nations-Population-Division. Accessed on: 20.8.2019.

World Health Organisation (WHO). (2003) Diet, nutrition and the prevention of chronic diseases. Technical Report Series 916, Geneva, Switzerland.

World Health Organisation (WHO). (2009) Monitoring Emergency Obstetric Care. A Handbook. WHO: Geneva, Switzerland. https://apps.who.int/iris/bitstream/handle/10665/44121/9789241547734_eng.pdf;jsessionid=B8A839EF25DAB6A A96817DD951D63238?sequence=1. Accessed on: 29.2.2020.

World Health Organization (WHO) and World Bank (WB) Group (2014) Monitoring progress towards universal health coverage at country and global levels. Framework Measures and Targets. Geneva: World Health Organization and International Bank for Reconstruction and Development/ World Bank; 2014 http://apps.who.int/iris/bitstream/10665/112824/1/WHO_HIS_HIA_14.1_eng. pdf. Accessed 15.4.2015.

World Health Organization (WHO) Health Topics (2019) Maternal Mortality (Overview). www.who.int/en/news-room/fact-sheets/detail/maternal-mortality. Accessed on: 20.9.2019.

World Health Organization (WHO). (2010) The World Health Report. 2010 Health Care Financing the Path to Universal Coverage. Geneva, Switzerland.

World Health Organization (WHO). (2013) Global Action Plan for the Prevention and Action Plan for the Prevention and Control of Noncommunicable Diseases 2013–2020. https://apps.who.int/iris/bitstream/handle/10665/94384/9789241506236_ eng.pdf?sequence=1. Accessed on: 13.6.2019.

World Health Organization (WHO). (2014) Making fair choices on the path to universal health coverage. Final report of the WHO Consultative Group on Equity and Universal Health Coverage.

World Health Organization (WHO). (2015) Tracking universal health coverage. First Global Monitoring Report. WHO and WB: Geneva, Switzerland.

World Health Organization (WHO). (2019a) Regional Office for Africa. Communicable Diseases. (Overview). www.afro.who.int/health-topics/communicable-diseases. Accessed on: 20.7.2019.

World Health Organization (WHO). (2019b) Global Dialogue on Partnerships for Sustainable Financing of NCD Prevention and Control. Meeting report, Copenhagen, Denmark, 9–11 April 2018. WHO: Geneva. https://apps.who. int/iris/bitstream/handle/10665/312289/WHO-NMH-NMA-GCM-19.01-eng. pdf?sequence=1&isAllowed=y. Accessed on: 20.7.2019.

Xiong Y, Cui Y, Zhang X. (2019) Pharmaceutical expenditure and total health-care expenditure in OECD countries and China: Bidirectional Granger causality on the basis of health level. Expert Review of PharmacoEconomics & Outcomes Research. https://doi.org/10.1080/14737167.2019.1605292.

Xu K, Evans DB, Kawabata K, Zeramdini R, Klavus J, Murray CJL. (2003) Household catastrophic health expenditure: A multicountry analysis. *The Lancet* 362(9378):111–117.

Xu K, Soucat A, Kutzin J, Brindley C, Vande Maele N, Toure H, Garcia MA, Li D, Barroy H, Saint-Germain GF, Roubal T, Indikadahena C, Cherilova V. (2018) Public Spending on Health: A Closer Look at Global Trends. WHO: Geneva. (WHO/HIS/HGF/HFWorkingPaper/18.3). Licence: CC BY-NC-SA 3.0 IGO.

Zhang T, Sidorchuk A, Sevilla-Cermeño L, Vilaplana-Pérez A, Chang Z, Larsson H, Mataix-Cols D, Fernández de la Cruz L. (2019) Association of cesarean delivery with risk of neurodevelopmental and psychiatric disorders in the offspring: A systematic review and meta-analysis. JAMA Network Open 2019 Aug 2: 2(8):e1910236.

Chapter 4

Equity lessons learned from pharmerging countries

The pharmaceutical industry is faced with challenges with regard to pricing and reimbursement. Patent expirations and changing market dynamics are driving forces of this environment (Karwal, 2006). The pharmaceutical sector was traditionally dominated by multinational companies from Europe and the United States, called "Big Pharma." Since the 1990s, Big Pharma has played a significant role in shaping the pharmaceutical industry, changing operating business models (Gautam and Pan, 2016). However, the pricing of pharmaceuticals and the high profits earned by Big Pharma companies have been of great interest, and it was stated that drug companies spend far more on marketing than on developing drugs (Deangelis, 2016). However, with the growth of emerging markets, they have become a key revenue contributor in the pharmaceutical market (Civaner, 2012).

The pharmaceutical market is dynamic and one of the most profitable trade sectors; it is actively moving the economy and has strong growth potential (Tannoury and Attieh, 2017). Despite global economic crises and governmental restrictions, the growth of emerging pharmaceutical markets is driven mainly by aging of the population, rising income levels, and the expansion of healthcare systems (Akkari et al., 2019). Emerging markets represent an exceptional opportunity for the pharmaceutical industry (Tannoury and Attieh, 2017). Changes in disease dynamics increase the need to improve accessibility and effectiveness of new pharmaceuticals. The development of new pharmaceutical products for treating chronic conditions such as diabetes is crucial (Even et al., 2017). Pharmerging countries are mostly developing nations, and they play a pivotal role in shaping and sustaining the growth of pharmaceutical industry (Akkari et al., 2019). Brazil, China, and Thailand are well known as pharmerging countries; they prioritize the manufacturing and use of unbranded pharmaceuticals (Lu et al., 2015). These countries have strong economic growth potential (Akkari et al., 2019), and new pharmaceutical companies that are emerging in countries such as China, India, Korea, and Brazil challenge the long-time leadership of the United States and countries in the European Union in the pharmaceutical market (Gautam and Pan, 2016).

In this chapter, pharmerging countries are examined with a focus on their experiences with healthcare reform to provide healthcare equity. First, the characteristics of pharmerging countries are described, followed by a discussion of their healthcare systems and equity experiences. In this regard, healthcare in Brazil, China, India, Russia, Thailand, and Mexico is examined.

Characteristics of pharmerging countries

Countries with emerging economies are also pharmerging countries (Civaner, 2012). Economists define emerging markets as countries with rising income. Leading emerging markets are Brazil, Russia, India, and China (BRIC) and Mexico, Indonesia, South Korea, and Turkey (MIST). Sales of the pharmaceutical markets in BRIC and MIST countries doubled in the 555 years between 2014 and 2019. As a result of increasing populations, increasing life expectancy, and growing prosperity, these countries increased their share of the pharmaceutical market by 20% (Tannoury and Attieh, 2017). A significant difference in disease dynamics has been caused by not only an increase in longevity and improvement in welfare status but also changes in lifestyle (Boles et al., 2017). These countries are following the same pattern as their Western counterparts with regard to the rise of chronic diseases, such as cardiovascular diseases and diabetes. According to predictions about diabetes and oncologic diseases, their incidences are expected to grow by 20% or more by 2030. As a result, pharmaceutical industries will continue to play a significant role in emerging economies (Tannoury and Attieh, 2017).

Historically, developments in the pharmaceutical industry have been shaped by developed nations in Europe and by the United States. Multinational Big Pharma companies, which have operated since the 1940s, have emphasized the importance of strong investments in research and development activities. This has resulted in the launch of numerous innovative medications, which have garnered high profits. Until the 1990s, prices and market acceptance were not officially controlled; as a result, these companies have shown strong growth potential (Akkari et al., 2019). During the 1990s, however, questions about the high prices of medications, competition from manufacturers of generic drugs, and more demanding regulations necessitated changes in marketing strategies. Under the threat of increasing competition, pharmaceutical companies began giving less importance to research and development activities and more to increasing their size (Akkari et al., 2019).

In 1994, the Trade-Related Aspects of Intellectual Property Rights (TRIPS) agreement was signed. This agreement is based on international standardization of intellectual property and imposes the same rules for all signatory countries. This agreement has had different effects in different countries; however; for example, growth opportunities in the pharmaceutical industry in developing countries have declined (Orsi and Coriat, 2006).

Brazil's agreement to TRIPS resulted in severe restrictions of learning by copying. This strategy is based on acquiring knowledge from pharmaceutically advanced countries, such as the United States and Japan, and it was to be used only for the production of medication with expired patents (Akkari et al., 2019). On the other hand, the adherence of China to TRIPS produced much more positive effects. China had provided for the manufacturing of products and processes in all sectors of its economy, including the pharmaceutical sector, since 1992; with the changes in its intellectual property system, China gained access to new technologies in the developed countries. After joining the World Trade Organization in 2001, China revised its protection standards:innovation is prioritized, and the number of intellectual patents increased at a rate different from those of other developing countries (Akkari et al., 2019). This strategy enormously increased the growth potential of the Chinese pharmaceutical market. Over the years, China has become one of the strongest pharmerging countries (Yu et al., 2010).

Many healthcare policy analysts agree that in developing countries, local pharmaceutical production can increase access to medicines and contribute to local economies (Dong and Mirza, 2016; Mackintosh et al., 2016; Mujinja et al., 2014; Russo and Banda, 2015). The market share of generic drugs differentiates Big Pharma from companies in pharmerging countries. India is one of the largest exporters of generic medicines at very low prices. Technology and various high-quality medicines are distinguishing features of the Indian pharmaceutical market. The Indian generic market is expected to reach US$55 billion in 2020 (IMS, 2011). China also represents one of the fastest growing pharmaceutical markets in the world. In particular, Chinese local generic drug manufacturers have increased their growth share exponentially: whereas it controlled more than 54% of total shares for generic drugs in 1999, that number rose to 62% in 2008 (Chhabara, 2010).

Figure 4.1 shows the market shares for generic drugs in developed and pharmerging countries. The United States is the leading market for unbranded generic medicines. European countries such as Germany, the United Kingdom, and France constitute the second biggest generic drug markets. The growth of the generic medicine market in China has been enormous, increasing from US$41 billion in 2010 to US$120 billion in 2015. Moreover, pharmerging countries such as Brazil and Russia also increased their generic market size considerably from 2010 to 2015 and have strong potential for increasing the market size of unbranded generic medicines (IMS, 2011).

The global healthcare community is increasingly advocating for the local production of pharmaceuticals in developing countries to promote technology transfer, capacity building, and improving access to medicine (da Fonseca, 2018) because local production plays a critical role in access to medicines (Bloom et al., 2019). The following sections provide overviews about pharmerging countries (Brazil, China, India, Russia, Thailand, and

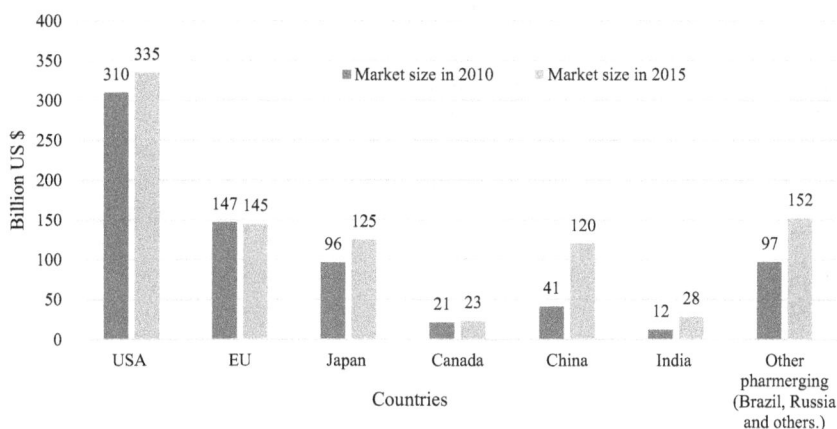

Figure 4.1 Generic market share in developed and pharmerging countries.

Source: The Global Use of Medicines: Outlook through 2015. IMS Institute for healthcare informatics. 2011. Retrieved from: www.imshealth.com/deployedfiles/ims/Global/Content/Insights/IMS%20 Institute%20for%20Healthcare%20Informatics/Global_Use_of_Medicines_Report.pdf. Accessed on: 10.7.2018.

Mexico) and their healthcare systems by focusing on healthcare policies that ensure equity in healthcare.

Brazil

The relationship between healthcare and local production of medicines and technology transfer is well exemplified in Brazil. Brazil has invested billions of dollars in the development of the pharmaceutical industry, including technology transfer agreements. At the same time, price control mechanisms are in place to meet health goals and to consider equity in the community (Flynn 2015; Shadlen and Fonseca, 2013). Brazil's experience suggests that innovative practices for technology and knowledge transfers can be created to ensure equity in the distribution of pharmaceutical prices. Moreover, it is believed that highly competitive pharmaceutical firms can collaborate with each other. Government support is critical for improving collaborations between pharmaceutical companies, which will improve the quality of pharmaceutical products. Healthcare policymakers and practitioners are trying to create a suitable environment for local production of medicines (da Fonseca, 2018).

The increase in the consumption of medicines in Brazil is one of the reasons for the emergence of generic drug programs. As one of the pharmerging countries, Brazil has a large share of the generic pharmaceutical market (Barra and Albuquerque, 2011). According to the Brazilian Association of Generic Drug Industries, there are 120 generic drug manufacturers in Brazil who are responsible for more than 3800 recorded medicines that were manufactured as a result of more than 21,700 commercial presentations. From an equity perspective, affordability of medicines for the general population is another reason for the increase in share of the generic drug market in Brazil (Bertoldi et al., 2019). The cost-related advantage of generic drugs is obvious for Brazil. It became possible to treat the most prevalent diseases with generic drugs, which cost as much as 35% less than the brand name products. Moreover, the statistical yearbook for the 2016 pharmaceutical market showed that 1.46 billion generic drugs were marketed in Brazil (Aquino et al., 2018).

Since 1988, Brazil has developed healthcare policies to achieve the objectives of Brazilian Unified Health System, which include provision of primary, secondary, and tertiary healthcare services and promotion of community participation (Barreto et al., 2014). The Estratégia Saúde da Família (Family Health Strategy) is a strong family healthcare program designed to achieve universal health coverage (UHC). It is also one of the biggest programs in the world for strengthening the primary healthcare system (Macinko and Harris, 2015). Under the Estratégia Saúde da Família, population coverage improved from 6.6% in 1998 to 63.7% (123 million people) in 2016.

There exist considerable differences in accessibility of healthcare between urban and rural parts of Brazil, as in most other developing countries (Hone et al., 2017). A significant goal of healthcare reform in Brazil is to enhance accessibility of healthcare services in rural parts of the country. In a program called Mais Médicos, implemented in 2013, approximately 18,000 doctors were hired in rural settings (Barreto et al., 2014; Santos et al., 2017). Despite success in improving primary healthcare services, inequities in the distribution of healthcare expenditures are considerable, in favor of rich households in Brazil (Mullachery et al., 2016). Moreover, a positive association exists between income and healthcare expenditure. Thus, inequities persist between rich and vulnerable populations in terms of financing of healthcare services. In addition, private health insurance is one of the causes of inequities in healthcare financing system (dos Santos et al., 2019). Nonetheless, the success of reform in primary care shows that similar efforts are necessary in the areas of secondary and tertiary care. More inclusive strategies of healthcare financing are needed to protect poor populations from high healthcare expenses (Barreto et al., 2014).

In Brazil, a program called *Farmácia Popular Program* (FPP) was launched in 2004. This is a government subsidy program for essential medicines. FPP allowed the establishment of a well-designed pharmaceutical information network in the country, which had important effects on the pharmaceutical market and sales of generic medicines. FPP promotes access to medicines for hypertension and diabetes in Brazil (Luiza et al., 2017). Moreover, this program reduces patient cost share, increases market sales volume of medicines covered by FPP, and increases the market share of generic drugs.

However, the sustainability of FPP is still questionable in the Brazilian healthcare system (Luiza et al., 2017). Compulsory licensing is another government strategy for controlling the cost of medicines in Brazil. This is not only a politically designed measure to achieve UHC but also a commitment at the local global level (Son et al., 2019).

Universal access to primary healthcare services has mostly been achieved by the Brazilian government. However, current equity analysis regarding specific healthcare services, such as maternal care, indicates inequities in Brazilian healthcare system in favor of wealthy citizens (Mullachery et al., 2016). These inequities are reflected mostly in quality of care and private health insurance systems (De La Torre et al., 2018). In view of the strong growth potential of the Brazilian pharmaceutical market, incentives to improve the generic drug market, government success in cost control, and UHC are advisable strategies so that Brazil can continue to be one of the strong pharmergers.

China

China implemented healthcare reform in 2009 to increase public healthcare financing, provide essential drugs, expand primary healthcare services, and achieve UHC by 2020 (Meng et al., 2015). The Chinese government implemented export-led growth strategies in healthcare as a development strategy in the domestic market (Fabre, 2015). In addition, the government established the Essential Medicines Program and paid primary healthcare providers to deliver a defined minimum package of public healthcare services (Yip and Hsiao, 2014). Despite the reduction of out-of-pocket (OOP) healthcare expenditures after healthcare reform, the effects of healthcare reform are still limited. The positive effects on outpatient services have been more notable than those on inpatient services. Healthcare policymakers must focus more on inpatient services in the next stage of reforms (Li et al., 2019).

The Chinese pharmaceutical market is driven by low-tech generic drugs. Generic drugs constitute 76% of the entire pharmaceutical market in China. Moreover, innovative drugs that are under patent protection account for only 4% of the market. The low-cost drugs constitute the largest segment of the pharmaceutical industry in China and are the domestic products under the most control. The Chinese pharmaceutical market is one of the most dynamic in the world. It grew 22% in 2010 to US$116 billion and ranked as the fifth largest pharmaceutical market in the world (Bioassociates, 2012; Chan and Daim, 2018).

China's healthcare reforms have increased healthcare expenditures. China has a great opportunity to develop market share and has enormous manufacturing potential (Rodwin et al., 2018). A relatively healthy environment for continuous innovation and drug patent protection provide significant benefits for the growth of the pharmaceutical industry in China. The benefits to the public also improved considerably. Despite these improvements, industrial and drug policy objectives in the pharmaceutical sector needs more attention (Chen et al., 2017). It is unclear whether pharmaceutical reform solves the problem of overly expensive healthcare services; increasing drug expenditures constitute a heavy burden on patients and are a major concern in China. Studies have verified that pharmaceutical reform failed to meet its goal of combating the sharp growth of drug and total healthcare expenditures (He et al., 2018). One of the shortcomings of Chinese pharmaceutical market is a lack of accessibility. Reassessment of the quality and efficacy of domestically produced generic medicine, coordination of price determination, insurance payments, and addressing medicine shortcomings are specific mechanisms to achieve sustainable and equitable access to expensive medicines (Sun et al., 2018). China has already achieved universal health insurance, and insurance funds have been the key source of financing of public hospitals. According to healthcare policy advisers, health insurance programs play a pivotal role in setting the maximum reimbursement prices in a systematic way, and incentives for cost-effective prescribing and use are needed (Sun et al., 2018).

One of the strengths of the Chinese medicine system is its ability to incorporate traditional medicine with modern treatments. The combination of traditional Chinese medicine with Western medicine benefits patients by improving their quality of life (Xie et al., 2018).

China has introduced a series of new policy regulations and has sought to increase international cooperation with healthcare reform (Wagstaff et al., 2009). Also, China promotes the entry of Chinese medicine into the international markets (Tang et al., 2018). Another advantage of the Chinese healthcare system is the number of international collaborations in drug research, whereas India is a pioneer in patent application and Brazil is a leader in scientific publications (Bennato and Magazzini, 2019).

The rising prevalence of chronic health problems, such as diabetes, increases the concerns for equity in Chinese healthcare system, and better planning for the future is necessary (Sun et al., 2017). China has the highest use of insulin cartridges and pens in the world. Market share of these agents exceeded 44% in China by 2012 (Lu et al., 2015). In other words, China was the fastest adopter of both insulin and oral hypoglycemic products. Chinese hospitals have derived a large proportion (more than 50%) of their operating budgets from drug sales (Sun et al., 2008; Yu et al., 2010). In China, to ensure the growth of pharmaceutical market equity and future sustainability of pharmaceutical system, better planning is needed for the pharmaceutical market. Existing evidence about availability, accessibility, and use of medicines shows that prices are lower at primary care facilities than elsewhere. However, the effects of healthcare reform on availability of healthcare services and appropriate use of healthcare services needs more attention in future studies (Xue-He et al., 2011).

Thanks to the motivation of ensuring equity in healthcare services, improving the quality of care, and enhancing the research and development capacity of the Chinese healthcare system, a strategy plan for the future was constructed. In China, the Healthy China 2030 program is a strategic action plan whose main objects are to encourage economic and social development, improve structural reform of the medical supply, and enhance national well-being and social stability (Tan et al., 2017). Four principles guide this plan. The first is health priority, whereby healthcare should be prioritized during the whole process of public policy implementation. The second principle is innovation; the healthcare industry should follow government leadership and accelerate reform in key areas of healthcare. The third principle concerns the importance of scientific development. The fourth principle emphasizes fairness and justice; that is, ensuring equity. This entails consideration of rural–urban differences with regard to equal access to basic healthcare services and the maintenance of public welfare (Tan et al., 2017).

India

India is one of the most populous countries in the world (Bhardwaj et al., 2018). In India, competition with regard to quality in branded generic and newly branded pharmaceuticals represents an opportunity for Big Pharma; the government encourages investment and yet remains protective of its manufacturing base for generic medicines (Rodwin et al., 2018). Research and development in the Indian pharmaceutical industry are intense; this is the distinguishing feature of the Indian pharmaceutical industry. Cash flow and past innovative output are positively and significantly related to the intensity of research and development. The global orientation of Indian pharmaceutical firms has been found to affect research and development activities considerably (Tyagi et al., 2018).

Since the mid-1990s, Indian pharmaceutical companies have emerged as leading suppliers of generic drugs to both developing and developed countries producing high-quality generic drugs (Mohiuddin et al., 2017). The Indian pharmaceutical industry is estimated to contribute 20%–24% of the world production of generic drugs. The sales volume of pharmaceuticals is also considerable; sales increased enormously from $100 million in 1947 to $12 billion in 2012 (Mohiuddin et al., 2017). Over the years, the Indian pharmaceutical industry has changed from importing to innovation of drugs. Changes and regulations in the Indian government's industrial and technology policies play a crucial role in shaping research and development in India. Basic and intermediate technological capabilities provide a solid base for development of competence in advanced innovative research and development (Kale and Little, 2007). Well-educated scientists, a well-established computer industry, and technological skill for the manufacture of bulk drugs and formulations enable Indian success (Joshi, 2003).

Moreover, institutional policies that promote collaborative research and development, as well as investment in infrastructure and human capital development, are driving forces of the development of advanced technology in India (Mohiuddin et al., 2017).

Inequities in the pharmaceutical market, exemplified by inaccessibility of over-the-counter (OTC) drugs and poor pharmacovigilance, are current problems in India (Panda et al., 2017). Health inequities, especially in low-income settings, are obvious. Studies of rural parts of the country indicate useful strategies to improve equity in the Indian pharmaceutical market. In India, sustained political commitment, supported with strong human resources, healthcare financing, and gender issues, is necessary to fight against inequities (Thomas et al., 2015). However, India is one of the biggest marketers of OTC drugs, which are the medicines that had been available only by prescription but later became available on a nonprescription basis (More and Srivastava, 2010). In India, most of the population is aware about OTC products; however, teenagers and young adults are less, so doctors' advice, brand names, pharmacists' advice, past experiences, safety for use, prior awareness, and friends' recommendations influence the purchasing of OTC products (Srivastava and Wagh, 2018). An effective pharmacovigilance system is needed, and the large number of recognized medical, dental, pharmacy, and nursing colleges in India can help provide the necessary human resources (Bhardwaj et al., 2018).

In India, despite national healthcare policies, inequity has remained high with regard to access to healthcare services. Moreover, public healthcare is in crisis from a divestment in public healthcare services and the global trend for privatization (Singh, 2008). New public management models, such as public–private partnership marginalize the poorest people. Global institutions such as the World Trade Organization influence national policies to benefit global business interests, but the results often have a detrimental effect on equitable access to healthcare services (Labonte, 2002). In this regard, incorporation of ethical principles into the healthcare policy-making processes is highly advisable for healthcare policymakers (Prasad and Sengupta, 2019).

India is a country with large social inequities, combined with rapid economic growth, and studies of healthcare inequalities are of interest to policymakers (Prasad and Sengupta, 2019). The number of studies of healthcare equity increased in India after 2005. Of these studies, 88% involved quantitative analysis, whereas 8% were related to health interventions or programs. Whereas early studies of healthcare equity focused on mortality, communicable and noncommunicable diseases, and nutrition, more recent studies have focused on noncommunicable diseases, mental health, risk factors for illness, and injuries (Bhan et al., 2016). Studies are mostly focused on women and children, but wealth and income are primary measures of equity (Story and Carpiano, 2017). Education and gender are other indicators that are commonly used in equity analyses of healthcare services in India. The number of studies about wealth, education, and regional aspects has remained steady over time; in contrast, the number of studies of gender disparities have been rising (Bhan et al., 2016). In India, large disparities in health indicators exist between rural and urban populations. Majority of Indians are impoverished and cannot afford high OOP healthcare expenses. They also suffer adverse consequences of poor-quality care. In this regard, India needs to rebuild its primary care system, while continuing research on acute and chronic diseases. UHC will be helpful in the restructuring of the healthcare system and will help modulate the increasing OOP costs of healthcare (Patel et al., 2015).

In India, researchers must focus more on rural and poor populations (Bhan et al., 2016). Healthcare equity can be improved in low-income settings. Information from rural parts of the country can enable useful strategies to improve equity in the Indian pharmaceutical market (Garg and Karan, 2009). In India, sustained political commitment, supported with strong human resources, healthcare financing, and the addressing of gender issues are necessary to curtail inequities (Thomas et al., 2015). Future studies in India should focus on healthcare inequalities by evaluating healthcare policy and programs from an equity perspective.

Russia

Healthcare system in Russia underwent significant transformations during the 1990s, with an emphasis on privatization under economic liberalization (Akindinova et al., 2016). In Russia, both public and private provision of healthcare services is available. UHC is one of the promises of the government; however, underfinancing an obstacle to universal access, and substantial inequalities in accessibility and quality of healthcare services exist across different regions and income groups (Dubikaytis et al., 2010). Moreover, marginalized groups do not receive services from the healthcare system and are not provided any benefits from healthcare policies. Russia's national healthcare system is thus in need of more reform (Cook, 2015).

In Russia, as in other countries, women live longer than man. In addition, in 2016, rates of mortality from lung cancer and cardiovascular diseases were higher in men. Of other former countries of the Soviet Union, Russia has one of the highest rates of alcohol-related mortality. A strong national healthcare policy would help lower the amount of alcohol use in Russia (Global Burden of Disease, 2016). A widely cited retrospective case–control study showed that, of Russians aged 15–54 years, 59% of deaths in men and 33% of deaths among women were attributable to alcohol consumption (Zaridze et al., 2009). On the other hand, there exist four resources in healthcare financing system in Russia: (1) general budget revenues (approximately 40%); (2) health insurance funds (25%); (3) OOP payments (nearly

30%) and (4) voluntary health insurance (Popovich et al., 2011). Private healthcare expenditures are higher than public expenditures. Of importance is that poor health outcomes constitute the significant reason for increases in private healthcare expenditures (Cook, 2015).

It is not known whether health outcome measurements are used in Russia or whether healthcare resources are allocated equally among the population (Khabibullina and Gerry, 2019). During the 1990s, the healthcare sector in Russia underwent a decade-long economic decline, and efforts were made to transform healthcare provision according to a market-based insurance model. During that period, public expenditures on health declined dramatically. Poorly designed healthcare reforms resulted in privatization and marketization (Cook, 2015). This led to political conflicts and disorganization of healthcare services. By the 1990s, key health indicators had worsened. The number of deaths exceeded the number of births by 11.2 million, and the population declined by about 700,000 per year. Infectious diseases reemerged and spread, and childhood immunization programs collapsed temporarily in parts of the Russian Federation. The economic crisis in the 1990s caused changes in income distribution and healthcare practices. These factors were barriers to universal access to healthcare services. Moreover, informal payments continue to exist, which is one of the shortcomings of the Russian healthcare system (Cook, 2015).

Between 2000 and 2010, the Russian healthcare system recovered in terms of financing, organizational success, and health outcomes. Economic growth between 2000 and 2007 provide resources to better plan healthcare expenditures and improve the quality of healthcare plans. The healthcare system had become more accessible, and demands for informal payments decreased (Popovich et al., 2011). The rise in power of Vladimir Putin strengthened the power of state, including governance of healthcare system. Putin focused on population decline and low birth rates, especially their negative effects on economic development and national security. He defined healthcare as a "priority task" in addressing the demographic crisis. However, Russia's healthcare system had already been characterized by obstacles and persistent problems (Cook, 2015).

Healthcare programs were devised to improve healthcare coverage. State-financed healthcare was increased significantly by the Program of State Guarantees for Medical Care (PSG). The PSG is a universal program developed to provide benefits by creating a single national pool. PSG is designed as a multilevel service delivery system with increased tertiary care, improved diagnostic capability in medical facilities, and reduced geographic variations in funding and services (Somanathan et al., 2018). In Russia, health is improved by PSG investments and reforms. Redistribution of fiscal resources help increase resource allocation to vulnerable groups (Vlassov, 2016; Somanathan et al., 2018). High public spending for hospital services improves access to inpatient care for poor patients, especially those who are elderly. Greater availability of diagnostic equipment at outpatient facilities is associated with increased access to tests and services. Healthcare spending directed toward primary care improved access to physicians and services in rural areas of Russia. Despite these improvements, limited PSG coverage for outpatient drug purchases means that OOP drug payments are among the biggest threats to financial risk protection (Somanathan et al., 2018).

Studies of equity effects have shown regional and rural–urban inequalities in healthcare coverage in Russia. Despite the growth in the Russian economy between 2000 and 2008, this improvement did not reflect the distribution of healthcare resources among the population (Tang et al., 2008). It has been stated that in Russia, inequality rose with rates of poverty in the 1990s and then rose still faster in the 2000s as rates of poverty declined. National survey results showed that by 2009, there was a high percentage of households whose members were not receiving necessary medical help or purchasing healthcare services because they lacked the ability to pay (Cook, 2015). High levels of inequalities are reflected by huge differences in the accessibility of healthcare services at different levels (Popovich et al., 2011). Private outpatient services cost one-third of average total household expenses while serving fewer than 4% percent of patients (Cook, 2015). Overall, healthcare expenditures are very income regressive, and so the proportion of expenditures on healthcare is higher for poor individuals. Russians in the top quantile of income seek medical help nearly 40% more often than do those in the bottom quantile. They spend twice as much in absolute terms, but the proportion of income spent is far less than the proportion of income spent by the bottom quantile (Blam and Kovalev, 2003, 2006). Most healthcare expenditures are OOP and are directed to the public sector (Cook, 2015).

Analysis of pharmaceutical market indicators has shown that the Russian pharmaceutical market grew by 6.7% (in ruble terms) in 2016. Moreover, the Russian pharmaceutical market grown mainly because of sales. In 2016, inflation in Russia slowed down to 5.4%, and medicine prices grew by 5%; these were the lowest inflation rates between 2016 and 2019. The market share of branded medicines is decreasing, and consumers are shifting to cheaper generics. In 2016, the average price of a branded drug package was ₽362, whereas that of generic medicine packages was ₽111 (Deloitte, 2017). The federal program of "pharmaceutical and healthcare industry development for a period until 2020 and thereafter" is based on four key principles: technological upgrading of the pharmaceutical industry; importing substitutions for drugs on the WHO (World Health Organization) Model List of Essential Medicines; launching of innovative domestic products; and stronger export potential of the pharmaceutical industry and availability of human resources with high capacity for innovation. For better access to medicine, the program Pharma 2020 specifies that the availability of local drugs on the WHO's essential drug list should increase up to 90% (Deloitte, 2017).

In summary, Russia needs to make better use of its resources, and a better healthcare policy is necessary to improve the health of individuals and the life expectancy of its population (Tagaeva and Kazantseva, 2017). Consistent healthcare policies must be sustainable for public health, for primary prevention, and to address healthcare inequalities (Shkolnikov et al., 2019). Moreover, in Russia, the decision-making approaches and technologies have not been used successfully to allocate healthcare resources; healthcare providers and nonmedical professionals must participate in these decisions. Much of the developed world demonstrates sustainable progress in health technology assessment, but Russian healthcare policymakers rarely provide empirical evidence; their experience with health technology assessment is still new, and they are just starting to study the valuation of health benefits (Khabibullina and Gerry, 2019). High-quality studies are needed, especially in regard to involving service users in the development of policies and strategies and in the planning and development of healthcare services (Semrau et al., 2016).

Mexico

Mexico's pharmaceutical policy is developing rapidly and in a state of ongoing implementation (Duenas-Gonzalez and Gonzalez-Fierro, 2020). Pharmaceuticals constitute one of the main industries, and administration of the pharmaceutical price regulation scheme is the responsibility of the Ministry of the Economy. Regulations of pharmaceutical pricing allow flexibility (Moise and Docteur, 2007). In Mexico, expenditures on healthcare services accounted for 6.2% of the gross domestic product (GDP). Pharmaceutical expenditures represent 1.7% of the GDP and 26% of the all healthcare expenditures (Organization for Economic Co-operation and Development, 2015). Access to medicines is realized through different social security schemes. Mexico's Ministry of Health provides direct access to medicines and healthcare to poor members of the population (Gómez Dantés et al., 2011).

Mexico is one of the Latin American countries in which decentralization of healthcare services has led to problems with access to healthcare, including medicines (Arredondo et al., 2005). Studies showed that in the late 1990s, only half of the medicines on the WHO Model List of Essential Medicines were available in public healthcare facilities. Scarcity of financial resources, inefficient procurement planning, and inefficient distribution are the reasons for the unavailability of medicines (Frenk and Gómez-Dantés et al., 2002). However, Mexico does not have a single and concrete national pharmaceutical policy. The Ministry of Health published a document, "Towards an Integral Pharmaceutical Policy for Mexico" ("Hacia una Política Farmacéutica Integral para México") that intended to serve as a basis for a national pharmaceutical policy; however, the policy described in this document has not been created (Moye-Holz et al., 2017). A strong capacity for innovation is essential for the development of pharmaceutical market, but there are barriers to innovation in the Mexican pharmaceutical industry. These barriers include insufficient funds for the discovery phase, unaffordable and limited capacity for performing preclinical studies, lengthy time until clinical trial approval, unclear policies for drug approval, and insufficient marketing (Duenas-Gonzalez and Gonzalez-Fierro, 2020).

Mexican healthcare reform has, however, increased the accessibility of medicines (Gutiérrez et al., 2014). A study about accessibility of financing and equity of pharmaceutical access revealed that for the poorest households without social security, medication expenses are higher than for the rest of the population (Salazar et al., 2016). For example, the cost of diabetes treatment with unpatented drugs is excessive. According to the study findings, the proportion of drug expenses in household income decreased by 11.79% in 1998 and by 11.59% in 2010. The introduction of generic drugs has affected wealth since 2010, and households spend more on medication (Salazar et al., 2016).

In Mexico, as in other countries, society is divided into rural and urban segments (Parker et al., 2015). In 2012, the Mexican government announced that the public health insurance, Seguro Popular, had achieved the goal of covering nearly 53 million individuals previously not included in the social security system (Nigenda et al., 2015). The objective of this program is to improve healthcare coverage and access to preventive services to otherwise uninsured people in Mexico (Rivera-Hernandez and Galarraga, 2015). Studies about equity effects of Seguro Popular have shown that older adults and people living in larger cities are better protected against excessive OOP healthcare payments than are their uninsured counterparts. Moreover, households in rural and smaller cities are faced with problems accessing healthcare. Thus, inequities do exist in Mexico, and poor households face financial risks in the Mexican healthcare system (García-Díaz et al., 2018). Further research is necessary to examine the distributive effect of coverage by Seguro Popular, social security, and other institutions providing health insurance (Parker et al., 2015). In other words, although this program has increased access to health insurance for the poor, inequalities in healthcare access and use still exist (Rivera-Hernandez and Galarraga, 2015).

Thailand

Thailand experienced economic crises and instabilities between the 1970s and 2000s. The 1997 Asian economic crisis caused Thailand's financial stock market to collapse. It took more than a decade for the GDP per capita to recover to the pre-1997 level (Julian, 2000). Economic performance was low in Thailand and average GDP growth was 3.5%. However, Thailand achieved upper-middle-income status in 2011 (WB, 2019).

Thailand's healthcare system is internationally known for its success in implementing UHC. Despite its low gross national income per capita, general taxation was used to finance Thailand's UHC without contributions from citizens (Tangcharoensathien et al., 2018). In 2001, Thailand implemented the Universal Coverage Scheme (UCS), a public insurance system whose aim was to provide universal access to healthcare services, including essential medicines, and to influence primary care centers and hospitals to provide healthcare services efficiently (Garabedian et al., 2012). Thailand is one of the first countries outside the Organization for Economic Co-operation and Development to have introduced a form of UHC (Ghislandi et al., 2015). UHC has had the following positive effects on health status of Thai citizens: first, UHC improved the likelihood that individuals, especially women, would have an annual checkup. Second, necessary hospital admissions have increased by more than 2%, and outpatient visits have increased by 13%. Moreover, there no evidence that UHC leads to an increase in unhealthy behaviors and reduction of preventive efforts. Inclusive efforts provide strong benefits for individuals (Ghislandi et al., 2015). A third positive effect is that extended coverage helps reduce childhood mortality rates and provides specific interventions such as antiretroviral therapy and renal replacement therapy that have saved the lives of adults. Efficiency, cost containment, and equity are the primary successful accomplishments of Thailand's healthcare reform (Tangcharoensathien et al., 2018).

The distribution of healthcare expenses between rich and poor members of Thai society is one of the determinants of equity in healthcare financing (O'Donnell et al., 2008). Moreover, poor households are faced with financial difficulties because of high costs of catastrophic healthcare (Xu et al., 2003). Successful experiences of developing countries in handling financial resource constraints have broadened the perspectives of Thai healthcare policymakers (Younsi and Nafla, 2019). In Thailand, people use inpatient services, especially at private hospitals. Use of services not covered by the UHC benefits package is expensive and leads to impoverishment (Limwattananon et al., 2007). Successful poverty alleviation strategies in Thailand, such as a comprehensive benefits package, with minimal copayment at the time of healthcare service, prevents catastrophic healthcare spending and protects households from being impoverished (Tangcharoensathien et al., 2018).

Medicines represent a key challenge to achieving UHC. Inclusive healthcare policies and regulations in the health insurance system have a strong potential to improve cost-effective use of medicines; however, the effect of inclusive insurance policies on household medicine usage in Thailand has not been studied extensively (Towse et al., 2004). Expanding healthcare coverage provides benefits to the entire Thai population, and access to medicines is increased. However, the UHC scheme does not seem to have increased the use of medicines for diseases that are typically treated in secondary or tertiary care settings or to have increased the market for generic drugs (Garabedian et al., 2012). Interventions related to health technology assessment are one of the positive outcomes of Thailand's UCS. Inclusion of new medicines and interventions into the benefits package enhances the efficiency of the healthcare system (Tangcharoensathien et al., 2018).

The UCS provides for sales of medicines for chronic conditions that are usually treated in primary care settings, such as diabetes, high blood pressure, and high cholesterol levels (Garabedian et al., 2012). Despite the increase in access to medicine, sales of medicines for severe diseases such as heart failure, arrhythmias, and cancer, which are often treated in secondary and tertiary settings, have not increased. This is consistent with the fact that the capitated payment system discourages referrals of UCS subscribers to higher level care (Hughes and Leethongdee, 2007; Damrongplasit and Melnick, 2009; Yiengprugsawan et al., 2011). To understand the effect of inclusive policies on individuals' treatment and medicine preferences, the experiences of other developing countries must be studied. On the other hand, under the capitated UCS payment system, sales of generic medicines, especially low-cost drugs, are expected to increase. In contrast to these expectations, study results emphasize that the majority of drugs for sale in Thailand are branded products, even though generic alternatives are available (Garabedian et al., 2012).

The expansion of healthcare coverage with a medicine benefit for the entire population, together with changes in the payment system and increased local manufacturing, has increased the per capita volume of medicines sold, thereby improving access to medicines in primary care settings in Thailand. Although health insurance coverage provide increasing numbers of benefits to the entire Thai population, future studies are necessary to examine long-term effects of UHC on medicine usage (Garabedian et al., 2012). On the other hand, the future of healthcare in Thailand depends on the development of precision medicine and genetic technologies. With an increasing ability to interpret genomic data, Thai physicians better understand their patients and are capable of managing genotype- and phenotype-related data (Shotelersuk et al., 2018). The cost effectiveness of precision medicine at the population level, accessibility and affordability of drugs, and specific treatments for rare diseases in low- and middle-income countries are essential equity concerns for healthcare policymakers from Thailand and other developing countries. Developing and developed nations must work together closely to improve inclusive, ethical, and cost-effective services in the field of genetic medicine (Shotelersuk et al., 2018; Thong et al., 2018).

The following chapters provide a brief overview of Turkey's inclusive health reform experience and measurement techniques and tools for studying the level of equity in healthcare services. After that, Turkey serves as a case country, and an equity analysis of the distributive pattern of pharmaceutical expenditures is performed in view of Turkey's experience with inclusive healthcare reform.

References

Akindinova N, Kuzminov Y, Yasin E. (2016) Russia's economy: Before the long transition. *Russian Journal of Economics* 2(3):219–245.

Akkari ACS, Munhoz IP, Santos NMBF. (2019) USA, Europe and pharmerging countriescountries: A panorama of pharmaceutical innovation. In: Mula J., Barbastefano R., Díaz-Madroñero M., Poler R. (eds) New Global Perspectives on Industrial Engineering and Management. *Lecture Notes in Management and Industrial Engineering*. Springer: Cham.

Aquino, S, Antonio Spina, G, Leitão Zajac, M, Luiz Lopes, E. (2018). Reverse logistics of postconsumer medicines: The roles and knowledge of pharmacists in the municipality of São Paulo, Brazil. *Sustainability* 10(11): 4134.

Arredondo A, Orozco E, De Icaza ED. (2005) Evidences on weaknesses and strengths from health financing after decentralization: Lessons from Latin American countries. *International Journal of Health Planning and Management* 20(2):181–204.

Barra ACG, Albuquerque I. de (2011) A decade of generic pharmaceutical policies in Brazil. *Journal of Generic Medicines* 8(2):72–75.

Barreto ML, Rasella D, Machado DB, Aquino R, Lima D. et al. (2014) Monitoring and evaluating progress towards Universal Health Coverage in Brazil. *PLoS Med* 11(9): e1001692.

Bennato AR, Magazzini L. (2019) Does regulation drive international research cooperation? Evidence from the pharmaceutical sector. *The World Economy* 42(4):1200–1223.

Bertoldi AD, Wagner AK, Emmerick ICM, Chaves LA, Stephens P, Ross-Degnan D. (2019) The Brazilian private pharmaceutical market after the first ten years of the generics law. *Journal of Pharmaceutical Policy and Practice* 12(18). https://doi.org/10.1186/s40545-019-0179-9.

Bhan N, Rao KD, Kachwaha S. (2016) Health inequalities research in India: A review of trends and themes in the literature since the 1990s. *International Journal for Equity in Health* 15(166):1–8.

Bhardwaj S, Verma R, Sharma R, Solakhia R. (2018) Pharmacovigilance: Dynamics in Indian pharma industry. *Indian Journal of Pharmaceutical and Biological Research* 6(1):30–33.

Bioassociates. (2012). Top pharmaceutical multinationals in China by investment. *BioMed Tracker*, 2012.

Blam I, Kovalev S. (2003) Commercialization of medical care and household behavior in transitional Russia. Draft paper prepared for Ruıg/Unrisd project on Globalization, Inequality, and Health. Unrisd, Geneva.

Blam I, Kovalev S. (2006) Spontaneous commercialization, inequality, and the contradictions of compulsory medical insurance in transitional Russia. *Journal of International Development* 18(3):407–423.

Bloom G, Katsuma Y, Rao KD, Makimoto S, Yin JDC, Leung GM. (2019) Next steps towards universal health coverage call for global leadership. *British Medical Journal* 365:l2107.

Boles A, Kandimalla R, Reddy H. (2017) Dynamics of diabetes and obesity: Epidemiological perspective. *Biochimica et Biophysica Acta (BBA) – Molecular Basis of Disease*. 1863(5):1026–1036.

Chan L, Daim T. (2018) A research and development decision model for pharmaceutical industry: Case of China. *R&D Management* 48(2):223–242.

Chen PP, Yuan CC, Hu YQ, Pei P, Jia S-Q, Wang EN, Xi X. (2017) Balancing industry and drug policy objectives in the pharmaceutical sector: The case of China. *International Quarterly of Community Health Education* 37(1):71–76.

Chhabara R. (2010) Cracking the Chinese Pharma Market. Reuters Events. Pharma. Market. Retrieved from: http://social.eyeforpharma.com/market-access/cracking-chinese-pharma-market Accessed on: 17.7.2014.

Civaner M. (2012) Sale strategies of pharmaceutical companies in a "pharmerging" country: The problems will not improve if the gaps remain. *Health Policy* 106(3):225–232.

Cook L. (2015) Constraints on universal health care in the Russian Federation. Inequality, informality and the failures of mandatory health insurance reforms. United Nations Research Institute for Social development. UNRISD, Palais des Nations, 1211 Geneva 10, Switzerland.

da Fonseca EM. (2018) How can a policy foster local pharmaceutical production and still protect public health? Lessons from the health–industry complex in Brazil. *Global Public Health* 13(4):489–502.

Damrongplasit K, Melnick GA. (2009) Early results from Thailand's 30 baht health reform: Something to smile about. *Health Affairs* (Millwood) 28(1):457–466.

De La Torre A, Nikoloski Z, Mossialos E. (2018) Equity of access to maternal health interventions in Brazil and Colombia: A retrospective study. *International Journal for Equity in Health* 17(43):1–11.

Deangelis CD. (2016) Big pharma profits and the public loses. *Milbank Quarterly* 94(1):30–33.

Deloitte. (2017) Russian pharmaceutical market trends in 2017. Deloitte CIS Research Center, Moscow.

Dong J, Mirza Z. (2016) Supporting the production of pharmaceuticals in Africa. *Bulletin of the World Health Organization* 94:71–72.

Dos Santos AMA, Perelman J, Jacinto PA, Tejada CAO, Barros, A. et al. (2019) Income-related inequality and inequity in children's health care: A longitudinal analysis using data from Brazil. *Social Science & Medicine* 224:127–137.

Dubikaytis T, Larivaara M, Kuznetsova O, Hemminki E. (2010) Inequalities in health and health service utilisation among reproductive age women in St. Petersburg, Russia: A cross-sectional study. *BMC Health Services Research* 10(307):1–7.

Duenas-Gonzalez A, Gonzalez-Fierro A. (2020) Barriers for pharmaceutical innovation with focus in cancer drugs, the case of Mexico. *Therapeutic Innovation & Regulatory Science* 54:342–352.

Even M, Zweekhorst M, Regeer B, Laing R. (2017) Baseline assessment of WHO's target for both availability and affordability of essential medicines to treat non-communicable diseases. *PLoS One* 12(2): e0171284.

Fabre G. (2015) The Chinese healthcare challenge: Comment on "Shanghai rising: Avoidable mortality as measured by avoidable mortality since 2000." IJHPM *International Journal of Health Policy & Management* 4(3):195–197.

Flynn MB. (2015) *Pharmaceutical Autonomy and Public Health in Latin America: State, Society and Industry in Brazil's AIDS program.* New York: Routledge.

Frenk J, Gómes-Dantés O. (2002) Globalization and the challenges to health systems. *Health Affairs* (Millwood) 21(3):160–165.

Garabedian LF, Ross-Degnan D, Ratanawijitrasin S, Stephens P, Wagner AK. (2012) Impact of universal health coverage in Thailand on sales and market share of medicines for non-communicable diseases: An interrupted time series study. *BMJ Open* 2(6):1–10.

García-Díaz R, Sosa-Rubi SG, Serván-Mori E, Nigenda G. (2018) Welfare effects of health insurance in Mexico: The case of Seguro Popular de Salud. *PLOS ONE* https://doi.org/10.1371/journal.pone.0199876.

Garg CC, Karan AK. (2009) Reducing out-of-pocket expenditures to reduce poverty: A disaggregated analysis at rural-urban and state level in India. *Health Policy and Planning* 24(2):116–128.

Gautam A, Pan X. (2016) The changing model of big pharma: Impact of key trends. *Drug Discovery Today* 21(3):379–384.

Ghislandi S, Manachotphong W, Perego VME. (2015) The impact of Universal Health Coverage on health care consumption and risky behaviours: Evidence from Thailand. *Health Economics, Policy and Law* 10(3):251–266.

Global Burden of Disease (GBD). (2016) Russia Collaborators (2018) The burden of disease in Russia from 1980 to 2016: A systematic analysis for the Global Burden of Disease study 2016. *The Lancet* 392(10153):1138–1146.

Gómez Dantés O, Sesma S, Becerril VM, Knaul FM, Arreola H, Frenk J. (2011) Sistema de Salud de México. *Salud Publica Mex* 53:220–232.

Gutiérrez JP, García-Saisó S, Dolci GF, Ávila MH. (2014) Effective access to health care in Mexico. *BMC Health Services Research* 14(186):1–9.

He Y, Dou G, Huang Q, Zhang X, Ye Y, Qian M, Ying X. (2018) Does the leading pharmaceutical reform in China really solve the issue of overly expensive healthcare services? Evidence from an empirical study. *PLOS ONE* 13(1):e0190320.

Hone T, Rasella D, Barreto ML, Majeed A, Millett C. (2017) Association between expansion of primary healthcare and racial inequalities in mortality amenable to primary care in Brazil: A national longitudinal analysis. *PLoS Medicine* 14(5):e1002306.

Hughes D, Leethongdee S. (2007) Universal health coverage in the land of smiles: Lessons learned from Thailand's 30 baht health reforms. *Health Affairs* (Millwood) 26(4):999–1008.

IMS. (2011) The global use of medicines: Outlook through 2015. IMS Institute for Healthcare Informatics 2011. Retrieved from: www.imshealth.com/deployedfiles/ims/Global/Content/Insights/IMS%20Institute%20for%20Healthcare%20Informatics/Global_Use_of_Medicines_Report.pdf. Accessed on: 10.7.2019.

Joshi HN. (2003) Analysis of the Indian pharmaceutical industry. With emphasis on opportunities in 2005. *Pharmaceutical Technology*. January. 74–94.

Julian CC. (2000) The impact of the Asian economic crisis in Thailand. *Managerial Finance* 26(4):39–48.

Kale D, Little S. (2007) From imitation to innovation: The evolution of R&D capabilities and learning processes in the Indian pharmaceutical industry. *Technology Analysis & Strategic Management* 19(5):589–609.

Karwal V. (2006) The changing competitive landscape in the global generics market: Threat or opportunity? *Journal of Generic Medicines* 3(4):269–279.

Khabibullina A, Gerry CJ. (2019) Valuing health states in Russia: A first feasibility study. *Value in Health Regional Issues* 19:75–80.

Labonte R. (2002) International Governance and World Trade Organization (WTO) reform. *Critical Public Health* 12(1):65–86.

Li J, Shi L, Liang H, Ma C, Lingzhong X, Qin W. (2019) Health care utilization and affordability among older people following China's 2009 health reform – Evidence from CHARLS pilot study. *International Journal for Equity in Health* 18(62):1–9.

Limwattananon S, Tangcharoensathien V, Prakongsai P. (2007) Catastrophic and poverty impacts of health payments: Results from national household surveys in Thailand. *Bulletin of the World Health Organization* 85(8):600–606.

Lu CY, Emmerick ICM, Stephens P, Ross-Degnan D, Wagner AK. (2015) Uptake of new antidiabetic medications in three emerging markets: A comparison between Brazil, China and Thailand. *Journal of Pharmaceutical Policy and Practice* 8(7):1-8.

Luiza VL, Chaves LA, Campos MR, Bertoldi AD, Silva RM, Bigdeli M, Ross-Degnan D, Emmerick ICM. (2017) Applying a health system perspective to the evolving Farmácia Popular medicines access programme in Brazil. *BMJ Global Health* 2:e000547.

Macinko J, Harris MJ. (2015) Brazil's family health strategy – Delivering community-based primary care in a universal health system. *New England Journal of Medicine* 372(23):2177–2181.

Mackintosh M, Banda G, Tibandebage P, Wamae W. (eds) (2016) *Making Medicines in Africa: The Political Economy of Industrializing for Local Health.* New York: Palgrave Macmillan

Meng Q, Fang H, Liu X, Yuan B, Xu J. (2015) Consolidating the social health insurance schemes in China: Towards an equitable and efficient health system. *The Lancet* 386(10002):1484–1492.

Mohiuddin M, Mazumder MNH, Chrysostome E, Su Z. (2017) Relocating high-tech industries to emerging markets: Case of pharmaceutical industry outsourcing to India. *Transnational Corporations Review* 9(3):210–217.

Moise P, Docteur E. (2007) Pharmaceutical pricing and reimbursement policies in Mexico. OECD Health Working Papers, No. 25.

More AT, Srivastava RK. (2010) Aesthetics in pharmaceutical OTC marketing. *SIES Journal of Management* 7(1):65–96.

Moye-Holz D, van Dijk JP, Reijneveld SA, Hogerzeil HV. (2017) Policy approaches to improve availability and affordability of medicines in Mexico – An example of a middle income country. *Globalization and Health* 13(53):1–10.

Mujinja PGM, Mackintosh M, Justin-Temu M, Wuyts M. (2014) Local production of pharmaceuticals in Africa and access to essential medicines: 'Urban bias' in access to imported medicines in Tanzania and its policy implications. *Globalization and Health* 10(12):1–12.

Mullachery P, Silver D, Macinko J. (2016) Changes in health care inequity in Brazil between 2008 and 2013. *International Journal of Equity in Health* 15(140):1–12.

Nigenda G, Wirtz VJ, González-Robledo LM, Reich MR. (2015) Evaluating the implementation of Mexico's Health Reform: The case of *Seguro Popular*. *Health Systems & Reform* 1(3):217–228.

O'Donnell O, van Doorslaer E, Wagstaff A, Lindelow M. (2008) *Analyzing health equity using household survey data: A guide to techniques and their implementation.* World Bank Institute. The World Bank. Washington, D.C.

Organization for Economic Co-operation and Development (OECD). (2015) Health at a Glance 2015: OECD Indicators, OECD Publishing, Paris. Retrieved from: http://dx.doi.org/10.1787/health_glance-2015-en. Accessed on: 2.7.2019.

Orsi F, Coriat B. (2006) The new role and status of intellectual property rights in contemporary capitalism. *Competition & Change* 10(2):162–179.

Panda A, Pradhan S, Mohapatro G, Kshatri JS. (2017) Predictors of over-the-counter medication: A cross-sectional Indian study. *Perspectives in Clinical Research* 8(2):79–84.

Parker SW, Saenz J, Wong R. (2015) Health insurance and the aging: Evidence from the Seguro Popular program in Mexico. *Demography* 55(1):361–386.

Patel V, Parikh R, Nandraj S, Balasubramaniam P, Narayan K, Paul VK, Kumar AKS, Chatterjee M, Reddy KS. (2015). Assuring health coverage for all in India. *The Lancet* 386(10011):2422–2435.

Popovich L, Potapchik E, Shishkin S, Richardson E, Vacroux A, Mathivet B. (2011) Russian Federation: Health system review. *Health Systems in Transition* 13(7):1–190.

Prasad V, Sengupta A. (2019) Perpetuating health inequities in India: Global ethics in policy and practice. *Journal of Global Ethics* 15(1):67–75.

Rivera-Hernandez M, Galarraga O. (2015) Type of insurance and use of preventive health services among older adults in Mexico. *Journal of Aging and Health* 27(6):962–982.

Rodwin VG, Fabre G, Ayoub RF. (2018) BRIC health systems and big pharma: A challenge for health policy and management. *International Journal of Health Policy and Management* 7(3):201–206.

Russo G, Banda G. (2015) Re-thinking pharmaceutical production in Africa; insights from the analysis of the local manufacturing dynamics in Mozambique and Zimbabwe. *Studies in Comparative International Development* 50(2):258–281.

Salazar REM, Pedroza JD, Trejo CZ, Acosta EJS. (2016) Access to medication in Mexico: Financing and equity. *Horizonte Sanitario* 15(2):63–68.

Santos LMP, Oliveira A, Trindade JS, Barreto ICHC, Palmeira PA. et al. (2017) Implementation research: Towards universal health coverage with more doctors in Brazil. *Bulletin of the World Health Organization* 95(2):103–112.

Semrau M, Lempp H, Keynejad R, Evans-Lacko S, Mugisha J, Raja S, Lamichhane J, Alem A, Thornicroft G, Hanlon C. (2016) Service user and caregiver involvement in mental health system strengthening low- and middle-income countries: Systematic review. *BMC Health Services Research* 16(79):1–18.

Shadlen KC, Fonseca EM. (2013) Health policy as industrial policy: Brazil in comparative perspective. *Politics & Society* 41(4):561–587.

Shkolnikov VM, Andreev EM, Tursun-zade R, Leon DA. (2019) Patterns in the relationship between life expectancy and gross domestic product in Russia in 2005–15: A cross-sectional analysis. *The Lancet* 4(4):e181-188.

Shotelersuk V, Tongsima S, Pithukpakorn M, Eu-Ahsunthornwattana J, Mahasirimongkol S. (2018) Precision medicine in Thailand. *American Journal of Medical Genetics* 181(2):245–253.

Singh H. (2008) Decentralization and public delivery of health care services in India. *Health Affairs* (Millwood) 27(4):991–1001.

Somanathan A, Sheiman IM, Salakhutdinova SK, Buisman LR. (2018) Universal Health Coverage in Russia: Extending coverage for the poor in the Post-Soviet Era. Universal Health Coverage Study Series. No. 37.

Son KB, Kim CY, Lee TJ. (2019) Understanding of for whom, under what conditions and how the compulsory licensing of pharmaceuticals works in Brazil and Thailand: A realist synthesis. *Global Public Health* 14(1):122–134.

Srivastava RK, Wagh S. (2018) Study of consumers' perception towards pharmaceutical over-the-counter products in emerging markets – India. *International Journal of Healthcare Management* 11(1):60–70.

Story WT, Carpiano RM. (2017) Household social capital and socioeconomic inequalities in child undernutrition in rural India. *Social Science & Medicine* 181:112–121.

Sun J, Hu CJ, Stuntz M, Hogerzeil H, Liu Y. (2018) A review of promoting access to medicines in China – Problems and recommendations. *BMC Health Services Research* 18(125):1–9.

Sun Q, Santoro MA, Meng Q, Liu C, Eggleston K. (2008) Pharmaceutical policy in China. *Health Affairs* (Millwood) 27(4):1042–1050.

Sun Y, Gregersen H, Yuan W. (2017) Chinese health care system and clinical epidemiology. *Clinical Epidemiology* 16(9):167–178.

Tagaeva TO, Kazantseva LK. (2017) Public health and health care in Russia. *Problems of Economic Transition* 59(11–12):973–990.

Tan X, Liu X, Shao H. (2017) Healthy China 2030: A vision for health care. *Value in Health Regional Issues*. 12C:112–114.

Tang H, Huang W, Ma J, Liu L. (2018) SWOT analysis and revelation in traditional Chinese medicine internationalization. *Chinese Medicine* 13(5):1–9.

Tang S, Meng Q, Chen L, Bekedam H, Evans T, Whitehead M. (2008) Tackling the challenges to health equity in China. *The Lancet* 372(9648):1493–1501.

Tangcharoensathien V, Witthayapipopsakul W, Panichkriangkrai W, Patcharanarumol W, Mills A. (2018) Health systems development in Thailand: Asolid platform for successful implementation of universal health coverage. *The Lancet* 391(10126):1205–1223.

Tannoury M, Attieh Z. (2017) The influence of emerging markets on the pharmaceutical industry. *Current Therapeutic Research* 86:19–22.

Thomas D, Sarangi BL, Garg A, Ahuja A, Meherda P, Karthikeyan SR, Joddar P, Kar R, Pattnaik J, Druvasula R, Rath AD. (2015) Closing the health and nutrition gap in Odisha, India: A case study of how transforming the health system is achieving greater equity. *Social Science & Medicine* 145:154–162.

Thong MK, See-Toh Y, Hassan J, Ali J. (2018) Medical genetics in developing countries in the Asia-Pacific region: Challenges and opportunities. *Genetics in Medicine* 20(10):1114–1121.

Towse A, Mills A, Tangcharoensathien V. (2004) Learning from Thailand's health reforms. *British Medical Journal* 328:103–105.

Tyagi S, Nauriyal DK, Gulati R. (2018) Firm level R&D intensity: Evidence from Indian drugs and pharmaceutical industry. *Review of Managerial Science* 12(1):167–202.

Vlassov VV. (2016) Russian experience and perspectives of quality assurance in healthcare through standards of care. *Health Policy and Technology* 5(3):307–312.

Wagstaff A, Lindelow M, Jun G, Ling X, Juncheng Q. (2009) Extending health insurance to the rural population: An impact evaluation of China's new cooperative medical scheme. *Journal of Health Economics* 28(1):1–19.

World Bank (WB). (2019) Thailand Overview. www.worldbank.org/en/. Accessed on: 10.10.2019.

Xie G, Cui Z, Peng K, Zhou X, Xia Q, Xu D. (2018) Aidi injection, a traditional Chinese medicine injection, could be used as an adjuvant drug to improve quality of life of cancer patients receiving chemotherapy: A propensity score matching analysis. Integrative Cancer Therapies. https://doi.org/10.1177/1534735418810799.

Xu K, Evans DB, Kawabata K, Zeramdini R, Klavus J, Murray CJL. (2003) Household catastrophic health expenditure: A multicountry analysis. *The Lancet* 362(9378):111–117.

Xue-He G, van den Hof S, van der Werf MJ, Guo H, Hu YL, Fan JH, Zhang WM, Tostado CP, Borgdorff MW. (2011) Inappropriate tuberculosis treatment regimens in Chinese tuberculosis hospitals. *Clinical Infectious Diseases* 52(7):153–156.

Yiengprugsawan V, Carmichael GA, Lim LY, Seubsman S, Sleigh A. (2011) Explanation of inequality in utilization of ambulatory care before and after universal health insurance in Thailand. *Health Policy and Planning* 26(2):105–114.

Yip W, Hsiao W. (2014) Harnessing the privatisation of China's fragmented healthcare delivery. *The Lancet* 384(9945):805–818.

Younsi M, Nafla A. (2019) Financial stability, monetary policy, and economic growth: Panel data evidence from developed and developing countries. *Journal of the Knowledge Economy* 10(1):238–260.

Yu X, Li C, Shi Y, Yu M. (2010) Pharmaceutical supply chain in China: Current issues and implications for health system reform. *Health Policy* 97(1):8–15.

Zaridze D, Brennan P, Boreham J, Boroda A, Karpov R, Lazarev A, Konobeevskaya I, Igitov V, Terechova T, Boffetta P, Peto R. (2009) Alcohol and cause-specific mortality in Russia: A retrospective case–control study of 48,557 adult deaths. *The Lancet* 373:2201–2214.

Chapter 5

Equity in health services in emerging markets similar to Turkey

Emerging markets have a high potential for explosive growth because of accelerating economic openness (Koepke, 2019). The BRICS countries (Brazil, Russia, India, Peoples Republic of China, and South Africa) represent the fastest developing emerging markets (O'Neill, 2015); and they have became powerful global competitors of developed nations (Denisov et al., 2019). This is despite their economies being predominantly agricultural-based. The BRICS's global economic reach reflects the healthcare and health spending moving from developed countries towards emerging markets (Jakovljevic, 2014). Successful health reforms in leading emerging markets have reshaped medical care expenditures (Jakovljevic, 2015). Thus, health reforms and the concomitant equity effects have become an increasingly relevant topic for health professionals and policymakers (Jakovljevic, 2014).

In addition to the emerging economies, the next 11 (N-11) economies, namely, Bangladesh, Egypt, Indonesia, the Islamic Republic of Iran, Mexico, Nigeria, Pakistan, the Philippines, Republic of Korea (South Korea), Turkey, and Vietnam have high growth potential and constitute a part of global share of healthcare spending. The joint contribution of these countries to the global health expenditures is substantially below that of the one of BRICS countries (Jakovljevic, 2015). The increasing burden of costly noncommunicable diseases and sedentary lifestyle is becoming more common in emerging economies (Jakovljevic et al., 2016), including Turkey (Kılıc et al., 2014). Moreover, increasing out-of-pocket (OOP) health expenses threaten the sustainability of medical care provided for their poor citizens.

This chapter will explain equity in health services by focusing on similar markets to Turkey in terms of level of development, geographic proximity, healthcare reform experiences, and significance of considering equal distribution of health resources. Further, specific policy suggestions will be offered to improve awareness of the equal distribution of health services.

Healthcare financing and affordability in the N-11 emerging markets

Global economic growth has been mostly driven by developing world economies. The most intensive part of global development consists of the BRICS nations in addition to the N-11 countries (Jakovljevic et al., 2016).

Equity in the provision of health services is an essential aspect of development for emerging economies. The timely definition of risks and improving equal distribution of resources is critical for the democratic provision of healthcare services and the credibility of health insurance systems (Das, 2009). Despite successful health reforms being implemented in these countries, BRICS countries are reshaping their medical care expenditures (Jakovljevic, 2015). Developed countries can be a role model for emerging ones; however, there is limited understanding about differences in long-term medical spending patterns between the Group of Seven (G-7) countries, traditional welfare economies, and the BRICS nations (Jakovljevic, 2015). Intercountry differences among the BRICS nations reflect health inequalities. A well-known example is the rural–urban differences in medical care affordability (Jakovljevic, 2014). Moreover, an aging population, a growing incidence of noncommunicable diseases, the high rural and urban migrations are valid health risks confronting all economies, especially developing nations (Watt et al., 2014). Increasing pharmaceutical spending is greatly related with an aging population and a high burden of noncommunicable diseases (Rancic and Jakovljevic, 2016). Thus, high OOP health expenditures affect the poor.

On the other hand, informal payments are a significant threat for the long-run viability of emerging economies (Leive and Xu, 2008). In other words, emerging countries still have a long way to go to design equitable health systems and provide essential and innovative care to the fastly growing middle-income class citizens (Das, 2009).

Considerable differences exist between the emerging economies in terms of urbanizations along with extreme regional differences in terms of access to medical care. Four out of the five BRICS countries share the challenges of rapid urbanizations (Ivins, 2013). China has pioneered high development capacity and output (Zhou and Leydesdorff, 2006). Additionally, the current evolution in medical spending is attributable to China (Han et al., 2008). Given that citizens of emerging countries are earning less money than their rich industrial counterparts, they have a high vulnerability to catastrophic health expenses. As such, there has been a sharp increase in OOP expenditures in the BRICS countries, from $67 purchasing power parity (PPP) on average in 1995 to $276 PPP in 2012. High informal payments threaten sustainable financing in emerging economies (Jakovljevic, 2015).

Pharmaceuticals are a costly aspect of healthcare. Thus, comparison of emerging economies by considering pharmaceutical market dynamics will elucidate understanding cross-country differences. As one of the emerging economies, Turkey has experienced an increase in importation of pharmaceuticals along with increased prices and expenditures, and increasing global regulations in the pharmaceutical sector (Semin and Guldal, 2008). Despite low drug consumption in Turkey compared to Western countries (Kısa, 2006), the level is growing, especially the consumption of antibiotics. Thus, Turkey has experienced both high dependency and financial resource constraints because of high level of drug consumption (Isler et al., 2019). In addition, Turkey's pharmaceutical industry is diverse; generic pharmaceutical products are being manufactured along with poor quality copies that have not been appropriately tested with regard to bioequivalence and bioavailability (Kisa, 2006). The domestic pharmaceutical industry has a low growth potential (Semin and Guldal, 2008). Moreover, in Turkey, cost-effective medical procedures and drugs are extremely limited, as they are in other emerging economies (Jakovljevic, 2015).

Providing universal health coverage is the ultimate objective of developing countries to provide health services for the poor and protect them from financial hardship (Wagstaff and Neelsen, 2020). Turkey has implemented significant reforms since 2003 to improve health benefits across different health insurance schemes. Incorporating Green Card users into the health insurance system, which represent vulnerable groups, is an essential part of unification of the system (Yardım et al., 2010). In 2005, social security beneficieries were able to access all public hospitals and pharmacies. In 2006, a pharmaceutical positive list across all health insurance schemes, including vulnerable groups, was integrated. With the 2007 Health Budget Law, benefits across all formal health insurance schemes were harmonized (Yardım et al., 2010). Despite these regulations and cost control strategies as regards health financing and affordability, the OOP health expenses remain high in line with other emerging economies (Rancic and Jakovljevic, 2016; TurkStat, 2018). Thus, despite Tuirkey's cost control regulations to protect poor populations and improve health services accessibility, there is still room to better understand the reasons of high OOP health expenses (Atun et al., 2016).

Other side of the coin, a considerable difference exists between low- and low-middle-income countries in terms of health spending levels (Dieleman et al., 2019). It is obvious that health expenses are relying heavily on OOP spending and development assistance (Mackintosh et al., 2016). In addition, comparisons by geographic proximity, population dynamics, sociocultural, economic development, and health system factors will enable the mitigation of increasing health expenses (Haakenstad et al., 2019).

Turkey enjoys a strategic geopolitic position along with strong cultural and economic ties with its neighbors (Onis, 2019). Moreover, Turkey has similarities with European countries, including a strong primary care system, aging population, and shortage of health workforce (Kringos et al., 2013).

Recently, Turkey has had a high refugee flux; therefore, to provide health services for Syrian refugees, a balance is needed in connectedness in housing them. This is critical to improve the health status of the people in the region (Willems et al., 2020).

The following section overviews healthcare financing and affordability for Southeast European nations with close proximity to Turkey.

Healthcare financing and affordability for Turkey's neighbors

Globalization challenges developing countries to better understand, coordinate, and manage population dynamics and health services. Moreover, the organizational apparatus of globalizations, such as intergovernmental or nongovernmental organizations, has been incorporated into the design and provision of healthcare services. However, scant evidence exists pertaining to global organizations's role in shaping the capacity of developing nations to highlight health equity (Tichenor and Sridhar, 2017; Forster et al., 2019). A generally accepted statement about health financing in developing countries is that nations with lower gross domestic product per capita spend more proportionally on medical goods, specifically, immunization and primary care services (WHO, 2002). Nevertheless, it is neccesary to consider each developing country's own dynamics (Jakovljevic and Souliotis, 2016).

Greece is one of the geographical peripheries of Turkey. Its access to healthcare services is largely determined by employment; those without jobs and their family members do not have comprehensive health coverage (Karanikolos and Kentikelenis, 2016). Variable economic parameters have a high potential to affect the dynamics of Greece's health sector. A severe financial crisis and recession occurred in Greece between the years 2007 and 2012, reducing its total healthcare and pharmaceutical expenditures (Jakovljevic and Souliotis, 2016).

Turkey and Greece apply the same control method for drugs, paying lower than the lowest reference price in the reimbursement system. Price comparisons, such as external reference pricing, with other countries is the primary criteria, and the ceiling price is determined on the basis of the lowest price in other countries (Atikeler and Ozcelikay, 2016). On the contrary, Greece is a regional refugee host country, constituting a key point of entry for the European Union (EU). However, there exists several problems in accessibility and utilizations of health services for immigrants due to sociocultural and language barriers. It is highly advisable to develop health policies to overcome financial restrictions associated with the lack accessibility of health services (Boutziona et al., 2020).

During the past decade, considerable policy changes have occurred to improve evidence-based decision-making in the health systems of developing countries. The World Bank has financed a formal Health

Technology Assessment (HTA) agency between the years 2005 and 2008. Budget funding was provided to large research projects to improve health economics in developing countries. Serbia has significantly benefited from these efforts (Novakovic et al., 2011), despite experiencing a serious financial crisis during the period 2007–2017 (Jakovljevic and Souliotis, 2016). In addition, considerable improvements have occurred in health technology assessment in Serbia, and thus it is necessary to develop cost containment strategies, but there is still a long way to go for full practical implementation in both Turkey and Serbia (Jakovljevic, 2013).

Croatia is another close neighbor of Turkey and a candidate country of the EU. The EU accession process broadens the vision of countries in the Western Balkans, such as Croatia and Turkey. Sizeable and credible incentives are offered to make structural reforms and to improve the citizen's welfare (Noutcheva and Aydın-Duzgit, 2012). Despite a low level of competitiveness, Croatia has experienced rapid economic development, placing it among high-income, non-Organisation for Economic Co-Operation and Development (OECD) economies. It has a formal HTA agency, with a healthcare funding experience similar to other Eastern Europe countries, such as shifting health expenditure from the public to OOP to attenuate financial deficits (Voncina et al., 2007). Systematic health evidence and official resource allocations are developing slowly and taking considerable interest from Croatian health policymakers (Jakovljevic, 2013).

Turkey has strong historical and cultural ties with Bosnia and Herzegovina (Mulalic, 2019). Expensive drug prices are rife in Bosnia and Herzegovina. Despite legislative frameworks include mandatory statements for cost-effectiveness analysis and local budget impact evidence for reimbursement of expensive drugs, they have not been enforced. A common approach is to lower price industrial offers for the domestic market (Markovic'-Pekovic' et al., 2010). HTA is inmature in Bosnia and Herzigovina, necessitating considerable time to improve systematic health economics evidence assessment (Jakovljevic, 2013). Rural–urban healthcare differences are palpable in Bosnia and Herzigovina as they are in Turkey. Hence, health policymakers should commit to improve health professionals' deployment into rural areas (Racic et al., 2019). Bosnia and Herzigovina are refugee host nations (Halliovich and Efendic 2019). Effective policies are neccassary to find solutions to political, economic, health, and social problems associated with migration (WHO Europe, 2019).

Albania is another strategic partner of Turkey. Political, economic, and defence relations between the two nations were redefined and strengthened after the Cold War. Turkey has supported Albania with investment in hospital groups (Xhaferi, 2017). In Albania, the health system was financed predominantly by the state budget and taxation. However, a huge informal sector and difficulties in collecting taxation are preponderant problems (Jakovljevic, 2013) in all developing countries including Turkey.

Despite structural problems of Albanian economy, including a strong informal economy, Albania has a young population with a healthy lifestyle (Mirmirani et al., 2008). The Albanian health system modernization project was started in 2008, which has provided HTA education for health professionals, sustainable health funding, and access to health services for vulnerable groups (Jakovljevic, 2013).

Kosovo and Turkey, middle-income countries, are also members and potential EU candidates (Tunali, 2017). Kosovo was one of the poorest countries in the region and invested heavily in its development. The dynamic socioeconomic changes after 1999 increased foreign investment to Kosovo's health sector (Buwa and Vuori, 2007). Kosovo has Europe's youngest population; however, key health outcomes such as life expectancy at birth and infant mortality are lower than the rest of the Balkans (WHO, 2010). In addition, OOP health expenses are high, accounting for 40% of total health expenses (Buwa and Vuori, 2007). The sustainability of health system financing is a long-term challenge, requiring growth in human resource investment and economic and technology assessment in healthcare. Maximizing health gains of the poor by carefully allocating scarce resources remains a preponderant objective of health policymakers (WHO, 2007).

Recommendations to build strong health systems in Southeastern Europe and Turkey

Health system funding and management is a great challenge for Southeastern Europe (Jakovljevic, 2013). Improving the quality and accessibility of medical care is a significant objective of health policymakers in these countries (MoH, Montenegro, 2011). Despite slow increasing cost awareness, the importance of health economics-based decision-making is improving. Socioeconomic inequality is increasing in the region, and it is becoming more difficult to deliver medical care in emerging markets with a rapidly growing demand for healthcare (Jakovljevic, 2013). Productivity is a major concern to improve quality of health services; however, Balkan health policymakers consider healthcare to be a consuming sector rather than a sector producing health. Thus, there exists little concern about health investments on productivity (WHO, 2007).

On the contrary, the frequency and length of hospital admissions in the Balkans are significantly higher than the EU average (Rechel and McKee, 2009). Not surprisingly, cost-effectiveness of medical products and the level of technology usage in health services have become increasingly important, with policymakers realizing the need for technology assessment in healthcare (Jakovljevic, 2013). However, number of health professionals specialized in HTA are limited to build evidence-based and less costly activities in healthcare (Jakovljevic, 2013). Additionally, hospital-based services constitute a large part of the services (Hysa, 2011). This means low affordability and a decreasing demand for necessary health services (Yamada et al., 2012). The worsening of the general population health in terms of neonatal mortality and life expectancy at birth are negative consequences of low accessibility to healthcare services (WHO, 2007). The pressure of traditional authorities and inefficiencies in the bureaucracy remain a significant obstacle to building more adaptive and accessible health policies for developing nations (Jakovljevic, 2013).

A number of countries in the EU have experienced difficulties in healthcare financing exacerbated by recession (Imasheva and Seiter, 2008). It is well-known that the primary financing source is tax collection for developing economies; however, this limits the income base to employed citizens. Problems occur in incorporating informal employment wages into the economic system (Jakovljevic, 2013). Thus, it is highly advisable to increase investment in healthcare, while pursuing practical applications about rational health spending (Jakovljevic, 2013). This will allow better affordability of health services and greater equity in healthcare accessibility, especially for vulnerable groups and an aging population (Garcia-Mochon et al., 2019). In addition, development of national guidelines on pharmacoeconomics and a localized HTA will help. These strategies are useful health and social policy actions to solve current obstacles in providing and funding medical care in the Balkan regions (Jakovljevic, 2013).

The N-11 countries consists of developing or newly industrialized nations. High infrastructure, urbanizations, energy, technology, and human capital are distinguishing features of these countries (Rancic and Jakovljevic, 2016). A high level of health expenditures and an aging population challenges health dynamics in these countries (Vancampfort et al., 2019). Each N-11 country confronts the heavy burden of population aging – the elderly's fight against chronic diseases is costly (Suzman et al., 2015). In addition, private expenditures on healthcare have recently increased, driven by OOP health spending. These factors are threatening the financial sustainability of population health in the next decades (Rancic and Jakovljevic, 2016); thus, providing strong physical and cognitive care for the elderly by considering cost dynamics is advisable for policymakers in emerging economies.

On the other hand, emerging economies are confronted with societal transformation, especially greater productivity and economic efficiency (Jakovljevic, 2014). High and costly noncommunicable diseases are a growing problem, and thus clinical efficiency and cost-efficiency is critical to fight against chronic diseases, such as cancers. So, policymakers need to consider reimbursement and affordability in their policy-making processes (Jakovljevic, 2014). Moreover, digitalizations of health services is on the agenda of health policymakers, which will ensure greater availability of health services and improved contact with health professionals (Mitchell and Kan, 2019). Increasing investment in digital health technologies is advisable to make health services more accessible for rural communities

(Mitchell and Kan, 2019). Comparison of health financing and affordability dynamics by considering geographic proximity factors is critical to build more affordable health systems (Song et al., 2018).

The emergence of the middle class and changes in individual consumption behavior in emerging economies is a driver of economic growth; and it is very much related to public health (Jakovljevic, 2014). In Turkey, changes in living standards and health behaviors parallel economic growth. Turkey is distinguished by a high level of consumption (Uner and Gundogdu, 2016). Rapid growth of the fast food industry, unhealty eating behaviors, and sedantery lifestyles increase the prevalence of noncommunicable diseases such as diabetes (Akbay et al., 2007; Kilic et al., 2014). Recently, Turkey has become a leader among European countries in diabetes prevalence (OECD, 2017). It is necessary to better understand health services accesibility and health behavior factors associated with diabetes and other chronic diseases in developing countries (Unnikrishnan et al., 2017). In this regard, providing patient education, counselling, and help in using digital technologies are all advisable to fight aganist chronic diseases and to better manage spatial health differences. Increasing collaboration between developed and developing nations will provide benefits to combat a high cost burden, and to provide equal health services for all.

References

Akbay C, Boz I, Chern WS. (2007) Household food consumption in Turkey. *European Review of Agricultural Economics* 34(2):209–231.

Atikeler K, Ozcelikay G. (2016) Comparison of pharmaceutical pricing and reimbursement systems in Turkey and certain EU countries. *SpringerPlus* 5(1876):1–8.

Atun R, Chaumont C, Fitchett JR, Haakenstad A, Kaberuka D. (2016) Poverty alleviation and the economic benefits of investing in health. Harvard T.H. Chan School of Public Health. Ministerial Leadership. Forum for Finance Ministers 2016.

Boutziona I, Papanikolaou D, Sokolakis I, Mytilekas KV, Apostolidiset A. (2020) Healthcare access, quality, and satisfaction among Albanian immigrants using the emergency department in Northern Greece. *Journal of Immigrant and Minority Health* 22:512–525.

Buwa D, Vuori H. (2007) Rebuilding a health care system: War, reconstruction and health care reforms in Kosovo. *European Journal of Public Health* 17(2):226–230.

Ciftci I, Tatoglu E, Wood G, Demirbag M, Zaim S. (2019) Corporate governance and firm performance in emerging markets: Evidence from Turkey. *International Business Review* 28(1):90–103.

Das DK. (2009) Globalisation and an emerging global middle class. *Economic Affairs* 29(3):89–92.

Denisov I, Kazantsev A, Lukyanov F, Safranchuk I. (2019) Shifting strategic focus of BRICS and great power competition. *Strategic Analysis* 43(6):487–498.

Dieleman JL, Micah AE, Murray CJL. (2019) Global health spending and development assistance for health. *JAMA* 321(21):2073–2074.

Forster T. Kentikelenis AE, Stubbs TH, King LP. (2019) Globalization and health equity: The impact of structural adjustment programs on developing countries. *Social Science & Medicine*. https://doi.org/10.1016/j.socscimed.2019.112496.

Garciá-Mochón L, Balbino JE, de Labry Lima AO, Martinez AC, Ruiz EM, Velasco RP. (2019) HTA and decision-making processes in Central, Eastern and South Eastern Europe: Results from a survey. *Health Policy* 123(2):182–190.

Haakenstad A, Coates M, Marx A, Bukhman G, Verguet S. (2019) Disaggregating catastrophic health expenditure by disease area: Cross-country estimates based on the World Health Surveys. *BMC Medicine* 17(36):1–9.

Halliovich H, Efendic N. (2019) From refugees to trans-local entrepreneurs: Crossing the borders between formal institutions and informal practices in Bosnia and Herzegovina. *Journal of Refugee Studies*. https://doi.org/10.1093/jrs/fey066.

Han Q, Chen L, Evans T, Horton R. (2008) China and global health. *The Lancet* 372(9648):1439–1441.

Hysa E (2011) Corruption and human development correlation in Western Balkan countries. *Euro Economica* 4(30):148–157.

Imasheva A, Seiter A. (2008) The Pharmaceutical Sector of the Western Balkan Countries. http://siteresources.worldbank.org/HEALTHNUTRITIONAND POPULATION/Resources/281627-1095698140167/PharmaceuticalsinWestern BalkansDP.pdf.

Isler B, Keske S, Aksoy M, Azap OK, Yılmaz M, Yavuz SŞ, Aygun G, Tigen E, Akalın H, Azap A, Ergonul O. (2019) Antibiotic overconsumption and resistance in Turkey. *Clinical Microbiology and Infection* 25(6):651–653.

Ivins C. (2013) *Inequality matters: BRICS inequalities fact sheet*. Oxfam Policy and Practice: Climate Change and Resilience 9:39–50.

Jakovljevic M, Groot W, Souliotis K. (2016) Editorial: Health care financing and affordability in the emerging global markets. *Frontiers in Public Health* 4(2):1–2. https://doi.org/10.3389/fpubh.2016.00002.

Jakovljevic MB, Souliotis K. (2016) Pharmaceutical expenditure changes in Serbia and Greece during the global economic recession (Original research). SEEJPH. doi 10.4119/UNIBI/SEEJPH-2016-101.

Jakovljevic MB. (2013) Resource allocation strategies in Southeastern European health policy. *European Journal of Health Economics* 14:153–159.

Jakovljevic MB. (2014) The key role of the leading emerging BRIC markets in the future of global health care. *Serbian Journal of Experimental and Clinical Research* 15(3):139–143.

Jakovljevic MB. (2015) BRIC's growing share of global health spending and their diverging pathways. *Frontiers in Public Health* 3(135):1–4.

Karanikolos M, Kentikelenis A. (2016) Health inequalities after austerity in Greece. *International Journal for Equity in Health* 15(83):1–3.

Kilic B, Phillimore P, Islek D, Oztoprak D, et al. (2014) Research capacity and training needs for non-communicable diseases in the public health arena in Turkey. *BMC Health Services Research* 14 (373) https://doi.org/10.1186/1472-6963-14-373.

Kısa A. (2006) Analysis of the pharmaceuticals market and its technological development in Turkey. *International Journal of Technology Assessment in Health Care* 22(4):537–542.

Koepke R. (2019) What drives capital flows to emerging markets? A survey of the empirical literature. *Journal of Economic Surveys* 33(2):516–540.

Kringos D, Boerma W, Bourgueil Y, Cartier T, Dedeu T, Hasvold T, Hutchinson A, Lember M, Oleszczyk M, Rotar Pavlic D, Svab I, Tedeschi P, Wilm S, Wilson A, Windak A, Van der Zee J, Groenewegen P. (2013) The strength of primary care in Europe: An international comparative study. *British Journal of General Practice* 63(616):742–750.

Leive A, Xu K. (2008) Coping with out-of-pocket health payments: Empirical evidence from 15 African countries. *Bulletin of the World Health Organization* 86(11):849–856.

Mackintosh M, Channon A, Karan A, Selvaraj S, Cavagnero E, Zhao H. (2016) What is the private sector? Understanding private provision in the health systems of low-income and middle-income countries. *The Lancet* 388(10044):596–605.

Markovic'-Pekovic' V, Stoisavljevic'-Satara S, Skrbic' R. (2010) Outpatient utilization of drugs acting on nervous system: A study from the Republic of Srpska, Bosnia & Herzegovina. *European Journal of Clinical Pharmacology* 66(2):177–186.

Ministry of Health (MoH) Republic of Montenegro (2011) Project for Improvement of Good Governance in Montenegrin Healthcare System: Strategy for Optimization of Secondary and Tertiary Health Care Levels with Implementation Action Plan. www.un.org.me/Library/Health/3a%20Strategy%20for%20Optimization%20 of%20Secondary%20and%20Tertiary%20Health%20Care%20Levels%20 with%20Implementation%20Action%20Plan.pdf.

Mirmirani S, Li HC, Ilacqua JA. (2008) Health care efficiency in transition economies: An application of data envelopment analysis. *IBER* 7(2):47–56.

Mitchell M, Kan L. (2019) Digital technology and the future of health systems. *Health Sytems & Reform* 5(2):113–120.

Mulalic M. (2019) Prospects for trilateral relations between Turkey, Serbia, and Bosnia and Herzegovina. *Insight Turkey* 21(2):129–148.

Noutcheva G, Aydın-Duzgit S. (2012) Lost in Europeanisation: The Western Balkans and Turkey. *West European Politics* 35(1):59–78.

Novakovic T, Tesic D, Stefanovic D, Medic G, Sovtic DD. (2011) Guidelines for pharmacoeconomic evaluation for Serbia. *Value in Health* 14(7), A358–A358.

O'Neill J. (2015) Building better global economic BRICs. Global Economics Paper No: 66. Economics; Research from the Goldman Sachs Financial Workbench. 2001.

Onis Z. (2019) Turkey under the challenge of state capitalism: The political economy of the late AKP era. *Southeastern European and Black Sea Studies* 19(2):201–225.

Organization for Eco-operation and Development (OECD) (2017) Health at a glance. OECD Indicators. www.oecd-ilibrary.org/docserver/health_glance-2017-en.pdf?expires=1582658612&id=id&accname=guest&checksum=B9599470D0 46852F8C532B4C72771235.

Racic M, Ivkovic N, Pavlovic J, Zuza A, Hadzivukovic N, Bozovic D, Pekez-Pavlisko T. (2019) Factors influencing health profession students' willingness to practice in rural regions of Bosnia and Herzegovina: A cross-sectional study. *Rural & Remote Health* 19(1):1–10.

Rancic N, Jakovljevic M. (2016) Long term health spending alongside population aging in N-11 emerging nations. *Eastern European Business and Economics Journal* 2(1):2–26.

Rechel, B., McKee, M. (2009) Health reform in central and eastern Europe and the former Soviet Union. *The Lancet* 374(9696):1186–1195.

Semin S, Guldal D. (2008) Globalization of the pharmaceutical industry and the growing dependency of developing countries: The case of Turkey. *International Journal of Health Services* 38(2):379–398.

Song Y, Tan Y, Song Y, Wu P, Cheng JCP, Kim MJ, Wang X. (2018) Spatial and temporal variations of spatial population accessibility to public hospitals: A case study of rural–urban comparison. *GIScience & Remote Sensing* 55(5):718–744.

Suzman R, Beard JR, Boerma T, Chatterji S (2015) Health in an ageing world—What do we know? *The Lancet* 385(9967):484–486.

Tichenor M, Sridhar D. (2017) Universal health coverage, health systems strengthening, and the World Bank. *BMJ* 358:j3347:1–5.

Tunali CB. (2017) An empirical analysis of the macroeconomic dynamics of innovation. In: Sener S., Schepers S. (eds) *Innovation, Governance and Entrepreneurship: How Do They Evolve in Middle Income Countries?* Palgrave Macmillan: Cham.

Turkish Statistical Institute (TurkStat). (2018) Statistical Year Book for the Year 2018. https://dosyasb.saglik.gov.tr/Eklenti/36164,siy2018en2pdf.pdf?0.

Uner MM, Gungordu A. (2016) The new middle class in Turkey: A qualitative study in a dynamic economy. *International Business Review* 25(3) :668–678.

Unnikrishnan R. Pradeepa R, Joshi SR, Mohan V. (2017) Type 2 Diabetes: Demystifying the global epidemic. *Diabetes* 66(6):1432–1442.

Vancampfort D, Stubbs B, Firth J, Smith L, Swinnen N, Koyanagi A. (2019) Associations between handgrip strength and mild cognitive impairment in middle-aged and older adults in six low- and middle-income countries. *International Journal of Geriatric Psychiatry* 34(4):609–616.

Voncina L, Dzakula A, Mastilica M. (2007) Health care funding reforms in Croatia: A case of mistaken priorities. *Health Policy* 80(1):144–157.

Wagstaff A, Neelsen S. (2020) A comprehensive assessment of universal health coverage in 11 countries: A retrospective observational study. *The Lancet* 8(1):e39–e49.

Watt NF, Gomez EJ, McKee M. (2014) Global health in foreign policy—and foreign policy in health? Evidence from the BRICS. *Health Policy Planning* 29(6):763–773.

WHO Europe. (2019) Health diplomacy. Spotlight on Refugees and Migrants. https://discovery.ucl.ac.uk/id/eprint/10081875/1/9789289054331-eng.pdf#page=181

WHO European Office (2007) for Investment for Health and Development: European Observatory on Health Systems and Policies, Health: A vital investment for economic development in eastern Europe and central Asia (2007). WHO: Geneva.

Willems S, De Smet H, Heylighen A. (2020) Seeking a balance between privacy and connectedness in housing for refugees. *Journal of Housing and the Built Environment* 35:45–64.

World Health Organization (WHO). (2002) Long-term care in developing countries: Ten case-studies. World Health Organization: Geneva, Switzerland. www.who.int/chp/knowledge/publications/Case_studies/en/. Accessed on: 26.2.2017).

World Health Organization (WHO). (2007) European Office for Investment for Health and Development: European Observatory on Health Systems and Policies, Health: A vital investment for economic development in eastern Europe and Central Asia, WHO: Geneva.

World Health Organization (WHO). (2010) Kosovo public expenditure review: World Bank report no. 53709-XK, poverty reduction and economic management unit, South East Europe and Baltic countries unit, Europe and central Asia Region.

Xhaferi P. (2017) The Post-Ottoman Era: A fresh start for bilateral relations between Albania and Turkey? *Australia and New Zealand Journal of European Studies* 9(1):42–62.

Yamada T, Chen CC, Smith J. (2012) Health disparities and health integration. *Health Behavior and Public Health* 2(1):21–37.

Yardım MS, Cilingiroglu N, Yardım N. (2010) Catastrophic health expenditure and impoverishment in Turkey. *Health Policy* 94(1):26–33.

Zhou P, Leydesdorff L. (2006) The emergence of China as a leading nation in science. *Research Policy* 35(1):83–104.

Chapter 6

Health reform in Turkey and inclusive policies

Turkey is a developing country; the Justice and Development Party (Adalet ve Kalkınma Partisi-AKP) is in power since 2002, and a significant part of AKP policies comprise inclusive policies in healthcare (Onis, 2015; Agartan, 2015).

AKP's comprehensive health reform program started in 2003, and one of the primary objectives of this program was to ensure "equity" in health services distribution (Akdag, 2011). Healthcare is a dynamic and popular policy area of the AKP government, and economic trends affect health policies and resource distribution decisions of policymakers (Yenimahalleli-Yasar, 2011)

This book chapter provides a closer look at the historical background of Turkish health reform, in the light of the general economy. After that, building blocks of AKP's health reform are discussed in detail. Next, the equity effect of health reform experience on different functions of healthcare services is explained. Lastly, it is underlined that there is a lack of knowledge and the increasing need to examine the equity effects of AKP's inclusive health policies on Turkish households.

Historical background of Turkish health reform

Turkey is one of the high-middle-income developing countries according to the WB country income classification. It is located in Europe and Central Asia (WB, 2018). The economic regime, the level of industrializations and political atmosphere shape the resource allocation decision of the governments (Storm, 2017). In this regard, the reorganizations of the healthcare system, redistributive policies and pharmaceutical sector reforms are discussed from the perspective of the industrializations process in Turkey.

A brief overview of Turkish neoliberal economy policies

Turkey has achieved significant industrializations in the post-war period. Following the transition to neoliberal policies, Turkey has been integrating into the global economy since the 1800s and 1900s. Economic growth gains momentum in industrializations drive. Turkey extended its imports and exports and diversified its international trade. European Union (EU) membership process and Customs Union provided significant benefits for the Turkish economy. The 2001 crisis is one of the crossroads of the Turkish economy (Onis, 2009).

The economic and social policies shape the extent and mechanism of income and wealth distribution. Thus, it is useful to briefly explain the background factors of the current economic status in Turkey. AKP is incumbent since 2002, and after more than a decade, continues to be so. AKP's economy politics are classified into three distinct periods. The first period is the post-2001 era, 2001–2002 is the period of post-crisis governance; 2002–2009 is neoliberal constructing and electorally competitive reform activism; and the late phase is the post-2009 period of policy stagnation and increasingly authoritarian political context (Acemoglu and Ucer, 2015; Gurkaynak and Boke, 2013; Onis, 2015).

Post-crisis governance was apparent between 2001 and 2002. There exists a close relationship with the International Monetary Fund (IMF) during that time. At the beginning of 2001, Turkey faced several financial crises. These crises caused the exchange rate to collapse, inflation to climb to 55%, and real Gross National Product to fall by 5.7% (Akyuz and Boratav, 2003; Dorlach and Savaskan, 2017). The Turkish coalition government employed Kemal Dervis as the minister of economy to combat the financial crisis, who was previously the vice-president of the WB. Kemal Dervis prepared an economy program to solve the problems of the economic crisis (Kutlay, 2019).

After coming into power in 2002, AKP applied a strong economic program of the coalition government. The distinguishing feature of the AKP government is its social neoliberalism. Redistributive policies in the areas of healthcare and housing played a significant role in strengthening AKP's power (Agartan, 2015; Dorlach, 2015). Existing literature emphasizes that Turkey's Mass Housing Administration (TOKİ) housing project is a strong predictor of the party's durability (Marschall et al., 2016). Strong political support sped up the Turkish economic growth between 2002 and 2009. This period also represents neoliberal constructing and electorally competitive reform activism (Dorlach and Savaskan, 2017).

The Turkish economy grew at almost 6% per capita (per annum)) –the fastest per capita growth since the 1960s (Acemoglu and Ucer, 2015). Strong political support is one of the critical factors of Turkey's economic success story. Moreover, the period between 2002 and 2009 is called as neoliberal constructing and electorally competitive reform activism (Dorlach and Savaskan, 2017). High-quality economic growth was observed during that time period, and productivity growth was one of the main achievements of this period. What is more important about this process is that the type of growth was multifactorial and total factor productivity growth. New and better companies emerged during this period (Acemoglu and Ucer, 2015). This positive economic and political atmosphere paved the way for a reformist atmosphere for specific welfare areas, such as healthcare.

Healthcare is one of the dynamic policy areas of the AKP government and one of the prior success areas of AKP policies since 2003 (Yenimahalleli-Yasar, 2011). AKP started to implement its comprehensive health policies with the introduction of the Health Transformation Program (HTP). The building blocks of this transformation program are to ensure equity in the health system. Strengthening primary healthcare, improving the accessibility of healthcare services, controlling increasing costs in healthcare, providing universal coverage, and improving quantity and quality of health personnel are the primary drivers of this reform (Akdag, 2011).

Health reforms were implemented since 2003. A single-payer system, family medicine system, adaptation of new payment system, and the redefinition of the role of Ministry of Health (MoH) as a major planning and service organizations were the significant reform implementations (MoH, 2003; OECD, 2008). Socializations principle of healthcare services is a long-term strategy in Turkey. The following section provides a historical overview of the health system reform experiences.

Historical overview of health reforms in Turkey

Turkey has a social health system since the Socialization of the Health Services Act in 1961. This system aims to provide health services for the whole population by considering equity. Building a social health system is one of the main objectives of this ideal. Governments of Turkey revised the socializations of health services ideal by implementing structural reforms. However, political instabilities put strong barriers on this ideal. Turkey was managed by military rule during the 1980s (Yenimahalleli-Yasar, 2011). In 1982, the constitution defined the role of government in the health system and stated that "everyone has the right to live in a healthy and balanced environment" (Constitution of The Republic of Turkey, 1982).

The 1990s witnessed coalition governments and liberalizations of policy, society, and finance in Turkey. Turkey's attempts to integrate into the global market began in 1980. According to the main economic growth indicators, the annual percent change of GDP in Turkey is 2.7 for the year 1988 and this increased to 78.2% for the year 1998 (Cizre-Sakallıoğlu and Yeldan, 2000).

The 1990s were the years of Turgut Ozal's economic legacy. Ozal's legacy encompassed several different dimensions not only in the economy but also in politics, culture, and foreign policy. Radical market-oriented economic reforms took place that were supported by a large segment of the electorate. Turkey's successful transformation to the neoliberal model of development was possible under the strong political leadership of Ozal (Onis, 2004).

The transition to the neoliberal model of development for developing countries like Turkey is undoubtedly difficult because this process is inevitable rather than voluntary. The balance of payment crisis is the factor behind the neoliberal policy preference of Turkey. Moreover, a supportive social and political atmosphere is essential for the further success of neoliberal policies. The late 1990s saw extensive involvement of the IMF in the Turkish economy becoming the principal actor in the banking sector (Onis, 2004). Ozal's policies were established to promote a probusiness, antilabor political atmosphere in the country. Party politics encouraged probusiness and antilabor political atmosphere (Bayirbag, 2013).

Under these policies, the Anatolian Tigers, which represented the conservative business community, were put at risk. They became vulnerable with an open economy. They were not strong enough to individually access the top executive state. Their response to this system was to build an organization named "MUSIAD" (the Independent Businessman and Industrialists Association – Müstakil Sanayici ve Işadamları Derneği). Some of the economic groups were apparently at a disadvantage under the effect of Ozal's neoliberal economic policies (Bayirbag, 2013).

However, these vulnerable groups became powerful after more than a decade when AKP came into power. Anatolian Tigers played a significant role in the success of AKP's high-quality economic growth between 2001 and 2007 (Acemoglu and Ucer, 2015). Therefore, the primary focus of neoliberal policies was to improve trade and economic growth rather than redistribution of resources and improvement of the welfare of the population (Vural, 2017).

Socialization of health services continued to be the primary ideal of the Turkish government during the 1990s (Yenimahalleli-Yasar, 2011). A National Health Policy Document was published in 1993. This comprehensive policy document comprised building blocks of HTP of the AKP government, which were implemented after it came into power. The main features of this document were: (i) family medicine system to improve primary healthcare, (ii) an autonomous secondary and tertiary health service system, (iii) establishing a more rational and performance-based payment system, and (iv) general health insurance system (National Health Policy Document, 1993).

Introduction of the Green Card scheme is another significant development in 1993. Benefits of Green Card users were extended under AKP's inclusive health policies between 2003 and 2008 (Aran and Hentschel, 2012).

The international integration of the Turkish health system with the membership of WHO in 1989 is another significant improvement of the health system in Turkey. However, health reform implementations did not find a stable political environment because of unsuccessful coalition governments (Yenimahalleli-Yasar, 2011). Onis (2009) suggests that the fact that coalition governments in Turkey have been unsuccessful should not necessarily imply that coalition governments are always prone to economic and political instability. Nonetheless, the Turkish coalition governments failed to succeed during the 1990s. Notably, socializations of health services and health reform objectives were not achieved during the 1990s.

Turkey faced a strong economic crisis during the years 2000 and 2001. The 2001 crisis is a kind of fiscal and balance payment crisis coupled with major structural problems in the banking sector. Cooperation with IMF, WB, and the EU helped to solve economic issues during that time (Onis, 2010).

After this process, Kemal Dervis prepared a strong economic program and AKP successfully implemented this policy after it came into power in 2002. Therefore, AKP's implementation of Dervis's program is one of the background factors for successful economic growth (Onis, 2009).

To sum up, the post-1950 history of Turkey is characterized by periodic economic crisis and restructuring of the policy process in the country. Elected governments adopted populist programs resulting in a financial crisis, which were resolved through military interventions (Keyman and Onis, 2007).

Those military interventions stopped popular distributional demands. When an economic regime is formulated in a top-down manner, it worsens social inequalities. Turkey is a specific example of a developing country where socioeconomic inequalities are geographically crystalized, and public policies tend to emphasize uneven development. Therefore, it is critical to remember that welfare politics and redistribution are the key components of national solidarity (Bayırbag, 2013).

Historical overview of the pharmaceutical industry in Turkey

Turkey has been criticized for its lack of transparency in pricing and reimbursement strategies in the pharmaceutical industry. And, lack of communication with the pharmaceutical industry is another criticized area (Varol and Saka, 2006). In Turkey, the development of the pharmaceutical industry parallels economic growth and industrializations (Vural, 2017). During the 1980s, privatizations and liberalizations of trade and services, including the health sector, gained prominence in Turkey (Semin and Guldal, 2008). After completing the Customs Union with the EU in 1996, Turkey began cooperating with the international pharmaceutical industry. This increased market sales along with original and licensed product sales and values (Vural, 2017).

In 1999, patent protection became mandatory, and an intellectual property regime came into force. Local pharmaceutical companies focused on generic production, enabling them to strongly cooperate with transnational pharmaceutical companies (Vural, 2013). During the first decade of the 21st century, the pharmaceutical industry was faced with a strong Intellectual Property Right environment, growing public healthcare expenditures, and favorable pharmaceutical control policies. During the period 2004–2008, pharmaceutical price and expenditure control policies were changed (Vural, 2015). A preponderant health reform objective, which began in 2003 is to promote the rational use of pharmaceuticals and medical equipment. Moreover, a national institute is planned to oversee the use of pharmaceuticals and reimbursement policies, while promoting the rational use of pharmaceuticals (Tatar and Kanavos, 2006). The first strategy to promote the rational pharmaceutical consumption is controlling the maximum prices of pharmaceuticals regulated through the External Reference Pricing (ERP) system, implemented by the Ministry of Health. The second strategy is a supply-side expenditure control, implemented after Turkey's centralizations of healthcare financing (Vural, 2015). The ERP system enabled the Ministry of Health to determine the prices of pharmaceutical products via a reference price level, which consists of a price level of a predefined set of EU countries, i.e., the "reference" countries: Spain, Portugal, Greece, and Italy for the year 2004. The price scheme was determined by using new criteria to define original and generic drugs; original drugs in Turkey would be set according to 100% of its cheapest price amongst the predetermined list of five EU countries (Vural, 2015).

In addition to price control strategies, the medical technology trade, consisting primarily of pharmaceutical and related items, remarkably increased during the period 1982–2003. Imports of finished products increased from 1.7% in 1982 to 48.9% in 2003 (Semin and Guldal, 2008). After the implementation of pharmaceutical price controls, the Social Security Institution (SSI) became Turkey's monopsonistic purchaser of health services and pharmaceuticals (Vural, 2015). Since 2009, the Turkish government increased the stringency of its pharmaceutical policy and implemented strong price control policies. High price cuts, compulsory discounts for both generic and patented drugs have affected the domestic and international pharmaceutical industry (Vural, 2015).

As a reminder, in Turkey, cost controls, price controls, and profit controls characterized pharmaceutical pricing during the period 1972–1984. In addition, profit controls and free pricing were preponderant in pharmaceutical pricing during the period 1984–2004. Reference pricing and international price comparisons have been implemented since 2004. Additionally, before 1984, pharmaceutical companies profit rates were high; while after 1984 under the effect of profit controls, pharmaceutical companies reported low profits. Between 1994 and 1999, on average they suffered losses (Semin and Guldal, 2008; Atikeler and Ozcelikay, 2016).

It is critical to note that in Turkey the number of pharmaceutical companies amongst the largest firms increased during the period 1979–2003 (Semin and Guldal, 2008). Implementation of a strict price policy since 2003 has drawn scrutiny from multinational pharmaceutical companies demanding relaxation of prices. However, the Turkish government has continued to implement a strict price policy due to electoral incentives (Dorlach, 2016).

In Turkey, pharmaceutical product users have been charged for drugs and medical devices as part of outpatient services since the beginning of the 1980s. In addition, charges for physician and dentist examinations for outpatient services was introduced following the health insurance system unification in 2008 (Yenimahalleli-Yasar, 2011). User charges generate inequalities and a lack of accessibility of health services, which in turn causes informal payments, usually in cash and made to physicians for medical and surgical services. Thus, in Turkey, 25% of total OOP health payments were informal (Tatar et al., 2007).

To conclude, globalizations obscures the domestic industries of developing countries such as Turkey. Turkey should establish and protect its own pharmaceutical industry (Semin and Guldal, 2008). Increases in costly noncommunicable diseases, such as cancers, threaten the future Turkey's pharmaceutical industry. In this regard, sustainable pharmaceutical price control strategies, better coordination of pharmaceutical companies, and the fight against informal payments are necessary to improve the efficiency of the pharmaceutical industry.

AKP's health reform

In Turkey, significant redistributive policies were implemented after AKP came into power in 2002. Significant reform in health system started since 2003 in Turkey to address the shortcoming related to financial protection, improving health outcomes, and providing financial security for financially weaker population groups (Atun et al., 2013). Healthcare sector became the primary playground of AKP government for more than a decade (Agartan, 2015).

Turkey's HTP began in 2003. In Turkey, AKP has continually maintained a strong parliamentary majority and long-term political stability since 2002. Over the years, the popularity of the AKP has increased in line with the effect of the high rates of economic growth it has delivered, averaging a 7.5% GDP increase each year (Onis and Bayram, 2008).

The consistent economic growth has provided a fiscal space to invest more in healthcare, and reorganizations of the healthcare system has become one of the major policy areas and focuses of the AKP government (Acemoglu and Ucer, 2015). Health system reforms resulted in significant health outcomes, provided financial protection for financially weaker groups, and controlled the cost in high-cost areas, such as the pharmaceutical sector. Improved financial protection diminished catastrophic health expenditures and contributed to reducing the level of poverty. Therefore, there is a positive relationship between increased health expenditures and economic growth in Turkey (Arisoy et al., 2010).

Poverty alleviation is one of the most significant global challenges (Whitehead et al., 2001). Health reforms influence access, utilizations of care, and financial protection (Wagner et al., 2018).

In the past two decades, international trends in market-based health sector reforms have been spreading around the globe. Although such attempts pose an apparent equity trend for European countries, low- and middle-income countries need attention in this regard (Whitehead et al., 2001).

Main tenets of AKP's health reform

The main components of HTP include the following areas: (i) coordination of all health institutions under one umbrella and coverage of all citizens with the construction of general health insurance; (ii) enhancement of primary care services and introduction of a family medicine model; and (iii) promotion of the private healthcare sector. Major objectives of the HTP are consideration of equality and equity in healthcare service financing and utilizations of healthcare services (Akdag, 2011). Therefore, socially inclusive policies are at the center of health reforms in Turkey.

Notably, healthcare system regulations positively affect healthcare outcomes. Under the effect of redistributive policies in healthcare, life expectancy at birth increased by 15.4%, from 65 years in 1990 to 75 years in 2009, reaching 78 years in 2015. In addition to objective health outcome indicators, subjective health outcomes, including patient satisfaction, have increased from 39.5% in 2003 to 75.9% in 2011 (Atun et al., 2013).

Primary care focused on universal care coverage implementation as a part of the HTP. This care coverage has contributed to improved user satisfaction in Turkey (Stokes et al., 2015). Protecting vulnerable groups from increasing health risks is one of the main parts of the health reform process in Turkey. The Green Card system is aimed at protecting the poor from increasing healthcare expenditures. As part of socially inclusive policies, the benefits of Green Card users have increased between 2003 and 2008. The budget for the Green Card program has expanded as the number of its beneficiaries have grown (Aran and Hentschel, 2012; Bugra and Candas, 2011; Erus et al., 2015).

Under the effect of health insurance inclusion strategies, the level of out-of-pocket (OOP) health expenditures decreased from 2003 to 2006. Establishment of the Social Security Institution (SSI) has served as a financial pooling and purchasing mechanism. Before the establishment of the SSI, there was an employment-based insurance system in Turkey (Akdag, 2011). However, reorganizations of an employment-based insurance system and solving problems related to the fragmented structure of the health insurance system began with the HTP. With these regulations, fragmentation problems concerning the structure of the health insurance system started to resolve. The Social Insurance Organization, the Pension Fund for the Self-Employed and the General Employees Retirement Fund for Civil Servants were merged under the SSI (Akdag, 2011).

Effects of AKP's health reform on different functions of healthcare services

Health reforms have significant effects on different functions of healthcare services. Under the impact of the health reform, individuals who had previously been unable to obtain treatment in university hospitals were only able to purchase insured drugs in designated pharmacies; however, following the reforms, they had access to the same hospitals and pharmacies as the civil servants (Buğra, 2018).

Contributory payments are implemented to control the increased use of health services. As part of reform, patients are obliged to pay contributory payments to have outpatient healthcare services and medication. The government stated that contributory payments are a kind of regulation to prevent unnecessary outpatient visits and excessive use of medications. However, the literature indicates that compulsory payments generate income-based inequalities in accessing healthcare services (Hazama, 2015; Yilmaz, 2013).

As a result of all these regulations, there is a considerable increase in general satisfaction with healthcare services. According to the Life Satisfaction Survey study results, general satisfaction from health services went up from 39.5% in 2003 to 75.9% in 2013 (TurkStat, 2011).

One of the successful implementation areas of HTP is the primary healthcare system. Family medicine model was implemented in 2004. This system provides various opportunities for vulnerable groups (Cesur et al., 2017). Improvements in primary healthcare system reflect an increase in primary care consultations per person. In Turkey, the total number of per capita visits to a physician increased from 3.1% in 2002 to 8.4% in 2015 (MoH, 2016). Assigning every Turkish citizen to a specific family physician is one of the key innovations of the family medicine system (Cesur et al., 2017).

Another significant health reform implementation is strengthening primary healthcare system with a pay-for-performance scheme in family practice. A recent study conducted by MoH examined the satisfaction of health professionals from the pay-for-performance system. Study results show that 20.9% of health personnel are in favor of the opinion that performance-based payment improves the quality of healthcare services. Moreover, health personnel think that performance-based payment increase unnecessary examinations and diagnosis (MoH, 2017). Therefore, even though the performance-based system has proven beneficial for health personnel, there is still room for improvement of primary healthcare services and quality of healthcare services (Hone et al., 2017).

Pharmaceutical expenditures constitute a large share of total health expenditures in Turkey. Thus, this is a significant component of health policy and health reform objectives. The pharmaceutical market is one of the broader policy areas of the AKP government (Vural, 2017). Turkey has experienced a substantial increase in total pharmaceutical sales from USD

2.5 billion in 2002 to USD 8.0 billion in 2012 consequent to improved access to healthcare after HTP that began in 2003. Thus, HTP necessitated a new pricing mechanism in the pharmaceutical market. AKP's major reform in the pharmaceutical price policy emerged in September 2009. Strict price regulations were implemented, and pharmaceutical prices were decreased substantially between 2009 and 2012 owing to strict pharmaceutical price regulations (Dorlach 2016).

Healthcare becomes focused policymaking area of AKP government

After more than a decade of health reform experience, healthcare has become a focus of Turkish policymakers. This active health policy atmosphere reflects the behavior of Turkish voters. Scholars suggest that the personal benefits gained from welfare spending increase the likelihood of voting for the incumbent (Kayaoglu, 2017). Therefore, healthcare reform has become a priority and an essential point on the social welfare agenda (Agartan, 2015).

Healthcare has achieved the highest level of satisfaction among the policies of the AKP government. When the voters were asked which AKP policies they were most satisfied with, the most prominent response was affordable access to healthcare services and drugs (Gür, 2011).

Scholars have suggested that the impact has been remarkably egalitarian as the reform has ended the occupational status-based inequalities in accessing healthcare and made it easy to access healthcare services (Yılmazi, 2013). However, there is a scarcity of knowledge through analysis of health expenditures, and health services use regarding the effect of health reforms on equity.

On the other hand, a common concern regarding Turkey's healthcare system is its high level of informality, which is one of the main problems of any health system. Notably, Turkey's healthcare system failed to provide universal health coverage mainly because of the prevalence of high level of informal payment (Yılmaz, 2013).

The changing direction of Turkish economy and need for equity analysis of redistributive policies

After more than a decade's experience of health reforms, the direction of the Turkish economy and health system structure has changed after 2007. Despite the continuation of economic growth trend since 2007, this growth is credit-based, consumption-led, and government supported. Thus, zero productivity growth exists, which does not help in leading Turkey to the next step of development (Acemoglu and Ucer, 2015).

Not only the quality of economic growth but also the direction of political focus has changed in Turkey after more than a decade. In recent years,

Turkey developed strong ties with the neighboring countries of the Middle East and Arab. Even though the EU is the major trading partner of Turkey, building strong relations with neighboring countries creates a new dynamism in economic growth. Turkey shares common culture and values with these countries. However, the difference between Turkey and these countries is that Turkey is poor in terms of energy resources (Austvik and Rzayeva, 2017; Onis, 2009).

After the stagnation of the EU and following the Eurozone crisis after 2008, Turkey's trade with the Middle East and Arab countries accelerated. Even though the image of Turkey has changed in the eyes of health policymakers moving to the Eurasian direction, Turkey is still a candidate of EU. The EU accession process is critical for Turkey for democratization, economic growth, pluralistic social and political directions. In this respect, it is necessary to ascertain that the current Turkish politics and building of strong ties with the Middle East and the Arab world is not contradictory but complementary (Onis and Kutlay, 2017).

Nonetheless, a comprehensive social security reform was necessary to reduce the pressure of this deficit on the public budget. Moreover, there are still concerns about transparency, accountability, and the independence of SSI from the government's political decisions (Wendt et al., 2013). Thus, providing institutional autonomy is necessary for the future sustainability of welfare distribution. Additionally, better strategies to control informal payments are required.

One of the recent health reform implementations in Turkey is that of the public–private partnership model in integrated health campuses (city hospitals). This model necessitates strong collaborations with the private sector, and huge investments are made into the health sector with city hospitals (Top and Songur, 2019). The scarcity of financial resources is one of the shortcomings of developing countries. Thus, it is strongly advisable to examine equity in Turkey's health market. Further examination of the pros and cons of the integrated health campuses project by determining their suitability, advantages and disadvantages of the model is necessary to consider cost, quality, and availability of healthcare services.

On the other hand, pharmaceutical expenditures are one of the costly areas of healthcare services. The growth potential of the pharmaceutical market is of significance in developing countries (Ridley et al., 2006). In Turkey, strict price policy is the main strategy implemented since 2009 to control pharmaceutical price increases. Additionally, improving generic drug use is supported by the government. Furthermore, the current pharmaceutical policy encourages "national pharmaceutical" production. Nonetheless, the current policy actions in the pharmaceutical market necessitate an effective high price strategy, strong communication channels with private pharmaceutical sector, and consideration of consumer's expectations (Dorlach, 2016).

Because healthcare is a popular policy area of the AKP government, continuous monitoring of the level of equity in the distribution of pharmaceutical expenditures is the only way to rationalize redistributive policies. Thus, the next chapter makes an overview of equity analysis techniques and after that an equity analysis implemented for the distribution of pharmaceutical expenditures in Turkish households by using index and curve approaches.

References

Acemoglu D, Ucer M. (2015) The ups and downs of Turkish growth, 2002–2015: Political dynamics, the European Union and the institutional slide. NBER Working Paper No. 21608.

Agartan TI. (2015) Explaining large-scale policy change in the Turkish healthcare system: Ideas, institutions and political actors. *Journal of Health Politics, Policy and Law* 40(5):971–999.

Akdag R. (2011) Turkey Health Transformation Program Assessment Report (2003–2011). https://dosyamerkez.saglik.gov.tr/Eklenti/2103,sdpingpdf.pdf?0 Accessed on: 1.8.2019.

Akyuz Y, Boratav K. (2003) The making of the Turkish financial crisis. *World Development* 31(9):1549–1566.

Aran M, Hentschel JS. (2012) Protection in good and bad times? The Turkish green card health program. World Bank. Policy Research Working Paper. WPS6178.

Arisoy I, Unlukaptan I, Ergen Z. (2010) Sosyal harcamalar ve iktisadi büyüme ilişkisi: Türkiye ekonomisinde 1960–2005 dönemine yönelik bir dinamik analiz [in Turkish] [The relationships between social expenditures and economic growth: A dynamic analysis intended for 1960–2005 Period of Turkish Economy]. *Maliye Dergisi* 158:398–421.

Aryeetey GC, Westeneg J, Spaan E, Jehu-Appiah C, Agyepong IA, Baltussen R. (2016) Can health insurance protect against out-of-pocket and catastrophic expenditures and also support poverty reduction? Evidence from Ghana's National Health Insurance Scheme. *International Journal for Equity in Health* 15(116):1–11.

Asfaw A, Jütting JP. (2007) The role of health insurance in poverty reduction: Empirical evidence from Senegal. *International Journal of Public Administration* 30(8–9):835–858.

Atikeler K, Ozcelikay G. (2016) Comparison of pharmaceutical pricing and reimbursement systems in Turkey and certain EU countries. *SpringerPlus* 5(1876):1–8.

Atun R, Aydın S, Chakraborty S, Sümer S, Aran M, Gürol I, Nazlıoğlu S, Ozgulcu S, Aydoğan U, Ayar B, Dilmen U, Akdağ R. (2013) Universal health coverage in Turkey: Enhancement of equity. *The Lancet* 382(9886):65–99.

Austvik OG, Rzayeva G. (2017) Turkey in the geopolitics of energy. *Energy Policy* 107:539–547.

Bayirbag MK. (2013) Continuity and change in public policy: Redistribution, exclusion and state rescaling in Turkey. *International Journal of Urban and Regional Research* 37(4):1123–1146.

Bugra A, Candas A. (2011) Change and continuity under an eclectic social security regime: The case of Turkey. *Middle Eastern Studies* 47(3):515–528.

Buğra A. (2018) Social policy and different dimensions of inequality in Turkey: A historical overview. *Journal of Balkan and Near Eastern Studies* 20(4):318–331.

Cesur R, Güneş PM, Tekin E, Ulker A. (2017) The value of socialized medicine: The impact of universal primary health care provision on mortality rates in Turkey. *Journal of Public Economics* 150:75–93.

Cizre-Sakallıoğlu U, Yeldan E. (2000) Politics, society and financial liberalization: Turkey in the 1990s. *Development and Change* 31(2):481–508.

Constitution of the Republic of Turkey-1982. https://global.tbmm.gov.tr/docs/constitution_en.pdf. Accessed on: 1.9.2019.

Dorlach T, Savaşkan O. (2017) The political economy of economic and social policy in contemporary Turkey: An introduction to the special issue. *Journal of Balkan and Near Eastern Studies* 20(4):311–317.

Dorlach T. (2015) The prospects of egalitarian capitalism in the global South: Turkish social neoliberalism in comparative perspective. *Economy and Society* 44(4):519–544.

Dorlach T. (2016) The AKP between populism and neoliberalism: Lessons from pharmaceutical policy. *New Perspectives on Turkey* 55:55–83.

Erus B, Yakut-Cakar B, Cali S, Adaman F. (2015) Health policy for the poor: An exploration on the take-up of means-tested health benefits in Turkey. *Social Science & Medicine* 130:99–106.

Gür A. (2011) "Adil Gür: Türk halkı, hükümetin en basarılı icraatı olarak sağlığı görüyor" [Adil Gur: Turkish People See Health Care as Government's Most Successful Accomplishment]. Interview by Omar Cakkal. SD: Sağlık Düşüncesi ve Tıp Kültürü Platformu (Platform on Thinking about Health and Medical Culture), May 18. www.sdplatform.com/Dergi/477/Adil-Gur-Turk-halki-hukumetin-en-basarili-icraati-olarak-sagligi-goruyor.aspx. Accessed on: 1.7.2019.

Gurkaynak R, Boke S. (2013) AKP döneminde Türkiye Ekonomisi (The Turkish economy in the AKP era) (in Turkish). *Birikim* 296:64–69.

Hazama Y. (2015). Health reform and service satisfaction in the poor: Turkey 2003–11. *Turkish Studies* 16(1):36–53.

Hone T, Gurol-Urganci I, Millett C, Basara B, Akdag R, Atun R. (2017) Effect of primary health care reforms in Turkey on health service utilization and user satisfaction. *Health Policy and Planning* 32(1):57–67.

Kayaoğlu A. (2017) Voting behavior of the youth in Turkey: What drives involvement in or causes alienation from conventional political participation? *Turkish Studies* 18(1):32–55.

Keyman EF, Onis Z. (2007) Globalization and social democracy in the European periphery: Paradoxes of the Turkish experience. *Globalizations* 4(2):211–228.

Kutlay M. (2019) Turkish Crisis and Aftermath (2001–2016). In: Kutlay M. *The Political Economies of Turkey and Greece*. International Political Economy Series. Palgrave Macmillan, Cham.

Marschall M, Aydogan A, Bulut A. (2016) Does housing create votes? Explaining the electoral success of the AKP in Turkey. *Electoral Studies* 42:201–212.

Ministry of Health (MoH). (2003) Türkiye Sağlıkta Dönüşüm Projesi Konsept Notu (Health Transformation Project Concept Note) (Ankara: Ministry of Health Project Coordination Unit).

Ministry of Health (MoH). (2016) Turkish Ministry of Health Statistics Year Book 2016. https://dosyasb.saglik.gov.tr/Eklenti/13160,sy2016enpdf.pdf?0 Accessed on: 28.1.2019.

Ministry of Health (MoH). (2017) Turkish Ministry of Health. Health Personnel Satisfaction Survey – 2017. https://sbu.saglik.gov.tr/Ekutuphane/kitaplar/SAGEMpersonelMemnuniyeti2017.pdf. Accessed on: 28.7.2019.

National Health Policy (NHP) Document. (1993) (Ulusal Sağlık Politikası Dökümanı) [in Turkish]. T.C. Ministry of Health. General Directorate of Health Projects. https://sbu.saglik.gov.tr/Ekutuphane/kitaplar/ulusalsaglikpolitikasi.pdf. Accessed on: 20.2.2019.

Onis Z, Bayram İE. (2008) Temporary star or emerging tiger? Turkey's recent economic performance in a global setting. *New Perspectives on Turkey* 39:47–84.

Onis Z, Kutlay M. (2017) The dynamics of emerging middle-power influence in regional and global governance: The paradoxical case of Turkey. *Australian Journal of International Affairs* 71(2):164–183.

Onis Z. (2004) Turgut Ozal and his economic legacy: Turkish neo-liberalism in critical perspective. *Middle Eastern Studies* 40(4):113–134.

Onis Z. (2009) Beyond the 2001 financial crisis: The political economy of the new phase of neo-liberal restructuring in Turkey. *Review of International Political Economy* 16(3):409–432.

Onis Z. (2010) Crises and transformations in Turkish political economy. *Turkish Policy Quarterly* 9(3):45–61.

Onis Z. (2014) Turkey and the Arab revolutions: Boundaries of regional power influence in a turbulent Middle East. *Mediterranean Politics* 19(2):203–219.

Onis Z. (2015) Monopolising the centre: The AKP and the uncertain path of Turkish democracy. *The International Spectator* 50(2):22–41.

Organization for Economic Co-operation and Development (OECD). (2008) Reviews of Health Systems – Turkey. https://read.oecd-ilibrary.org/social-issues-migration-health/oecd-reviews-of-health-systems-turkey-2008_9789264051096-en#page3. Accessed on: 20.6.2019.

Ozgen H, Sahin B, Belli P, Tatar M, Berman P. (2009) Predictors of informal health payments: The example from Turkey. *Journal of Medical Systems* 34(3):387–396.

Ridley DB, Grabowski HG, Moe JL. (2006) Developing drugs for developing countries. *Health Affairs* (Millwood) 25(2):313–324.

Semin S, Guldal D. (2008) Globalization of the pharmaceutical industry and the growing dependency of developing countries: The case of Turkey. *International Journal of Health Services* 38(2):379–398.

Stokes J, Gurol-Urgancı I, Hone T, Atun R. (2015) Effect of health system reforms in Turkey on user satisfaction. *Journal of Global Health* 5(2):1–10.

Storm S. (2017) The political economy of industrialization. Development and Change. doi: 10.1111/dech.12281.

Tatar M, Kanavos P. (2006) Health care reform in Turkey. *Eurohealth* 12(1):20–22.

Tatar M, Ozgen H, Sahin B, Belli P, Berman P. (2007) Informal payments in the health sector: A case study from Turkey. *Health Affairs* (Millwood) 26(4):1029–1039.

Top M, Songur C. (2019) Opinions and evaluations of stakeholders in the implementation of the public-private partnership (PPP) model in integrated health campuses (city hospitals) in Turkey. *International Journal of Health Planning and Management.* 34(1):e241–e263. https://doi.org/10.1002/hpm.2644. Accessed on: 20.2.2019.

Turkish Statistical Institute (TurkStat). (2011). www.turkstat.gov.tr/PreTabloArama.do?metod=search&araType=hb_x Accessed on: 20.2.2019.

Varol N, Saka O. (2006) Health care and pharmaceutical policies in Turkey after 2003. *Eurohealth* 14(4):29–32.

Vural IE. (2013) Neoliberalism, Intellectual Property Rights and the Turkish Pharmaceutical Industry in the 2000s. In: Löfgren H., Williams O.D. (eds) *The New Political Economy of Pharmaceuticals*. International Political Economy Series. Palgrave Macmillan: London.

Vural IE. (2015) Politics, reforms, and regulation of pharma prices and expenditures in Turkey over the 2000s. In: Zaheer-Ud-Din Babar (eds) *Pharmaceutical Prices in the 21st Century*. Springer International: Cham, 2015, 267–296.

Vural IE. (2017) Financialisation in health care: An analysis of private equity fund investments in Turkey. *Social Science & Medicine* 187:276–286.

Wagner N, Quimbo S, Shimkhada R, Peabody J. (2018) Does health insurance coverage or improved quality protect better against out-of-pocket payments? Experimental evidence from Philippines. *Social Science & Medicine* 204:51–58.

Wendt C, Agartan TI, Kaminska ME. (2013) Social health insurance without corporate actors: Changes in self-regulation in Germany, Poland and Turkey. *Social Science & Medicine* 86:88–95.

Whitehead M, Dahlgren G, Evans T. (2001) Equity and health sector reforms: Can low-income countries escape the medical poverty trap? *The Lancet* 358(9284):833–836.

World Bank (WB). (2018) Country and Leading Groups. https://datahelpdesk.worldbank.org/knowledgebase/articles/906519-world-bank-country-and-lending-groups. Accessed on: 24.1.2019.

Yenimahalleli Yasar G. (2011) 'Health transformation programme' in Turkey: An assessment. *International Journal of Health Planning and Management* 26(2):110–133.

Yılmaz V. (2013) Changing origins of inequalities in access to health care services in turkey: From occupational status to income. *New Perspectives on Turkey* 48:55–77.

Chapter 7

Measurement of the level of equity in healthcare services

Measurement of the level of equity is an essential step in understanding the level of equity in the distribution of healthcare services (O'Donnell et al., 2008). A considerable number of approaches and measurement tools for measuring the level of equity exist in the literature (Xu et al., 2003). Undoubtedly, this is a technical issue, and developed countries are at an advantage than developing and underdeveloped countries. In this regard, sharing of data and knowledge between developed and developing countries is essential for uncovering inequities in healthcare services and protecting vulnerable groups (Binagwaho et al., 2013; WHO, 2013).

This chapter focuses on the equity measurement techniques in healthcare services. First, the index approaches are explained, which are summary indicators of the level of equity. Subsequently, the curve approach is explained with illustration.

Equity measurement in healthcare services

Considerable attention has been focused on the conceptual and empirical issues of measuring the fairness of household financial contributions to the health system (Xu et al., 2003). The World Health Organization (WHO) has stated that fairness in health system design will be possible by organizing an equal burden of payments and providing equal benefits in terms of healthcare services in the community (WHO, 2010). Thus, an equal burden of payments and health benefits is crucial for the financial sustainability of the health system (Cylus et al., 2019).

Indices are summary measures of equality in healthcare. These are traditional ways of measuring the distributive pattern of out-of-pocket (OOP) health expenditures. Combination of index and curve approaches enables seeing the bigger picture of the burden of OOP health expenditures (Wagstaff et al., 1989).

In other words, index and curve approaches complement each other and make it easy to determine whether the burden of OOP health expenditures is on the shoulders of the rich or poor populations (Wagstaff et al., 2011).

The natural and well-known way for assessing redistributive impact is to compute the difference between Gini coefficients for pre- and postpayment income. Notably, several factors affect the redistributive pattern of health expenditures. The effect of the average proportion of income spent on healthcare is one of these factors (O'Donnell et al., 2008).

The progressivity of the healthcare financing system is the second factor. The extent to which households with similar incomes are treated unequally and the extent of any reranking in the move from the prepayment income distribution to the postpayment income distribution is the final factor that affects the redistributive pattern of health expenditures (Aronson et al., 1994).

Health policymakers and planners need to design a health system that will enable households to contribute equally to the health financing system proportional to their income level (O'Donnell et al., 2008). Index and curve approaches are commonly used by policymakers and health planners to examine the redistributive pattern of OOP health expenditures and different functions of health expenditures, such as pharmaceutical products and medical devices in any country. These approaches enable to make cross-country comparisons regarding equity by considering the distribution of health and economic resources (Xu et al., 2003; Wagstaff et al., 2011). The following section gives an overview of the commonly used index and curve approaches to analyze the redistributive pattern of OOP health expenditures.

Index approaches

Index and curve approaches are traditional methods used in the measurement of inequity in healthcare. Various indices have been applied to different health variables as a measure of inequity in the literature (Erreygers et al., 2012). Common index approaches are summarized in the following section.

Traditional ways of measuring inequalities

Gini and concentration indices are the traditional and well-known measures of inequalities in the literature. Among these indices, the Gini index is one of the popular measures of income inequality in health economics. This index calculates the distribution of income between individuals and deviates from fully equal income distribution in the economy. Index values measure changes in values between 0 and 1, with the value of 1 representing perfect inequality (O'Donnell et al., 2008).

The concentration index is a measure of the degree of socioeconomic inequality in health variables (Wagstaff et al., 1989). It has been used for measuring and comparing the degree of socioeconomic-related inequality in healthcare (Wagstaff 2000). The concentration index is defined referring to the concentration curve and the line of equality (the 45-degree line). If no socioeconomic-related inequality exists, the concentration index takes a score of 0 (Wagstaff et al., 2011). Therefore, the index is bounded between –1 and 1. The index score is bounded between –1 and 1:

$$C = \frac{2}{\mu} \operatorname{cov}(h, r) \tag{7.1}$$

Changing income inequality affects the concentration index measure of income-related health inequality. The concentration index summarizes information from the concentration curve and can do so only through the imposition of value judgments about the weight given to inequality at different points in the income distribution (Wagstaff et al., 2011).

There is a vast literature on measuring inequalities by considering income level differences of individuals, especially in the context of healthcare services. The family of entropy indices is another way of measuring inequalities. Theil (T) and Mean Logarithmic Deviation (MLD) are well-known examples of entropy indices (Xu et al., 2003). The following section gives more details regarding entropy indices.

Entropy indices

Entropy originates from the notion of information theory. Entropy indices are the measures that examine the value of various events with regard to their likelihood of occurrence. These indices are measuring inequality, including T and MLD. T measures the difference between the maximum and the expected value of a variable. This index assesses the value of different events to their likelihood of occurrence (Xu et al., 2003). T measures the difference between the maximum and the expected value of a variable, which is shown in equation (7.2). In this equation, "n" stands for independent events and each of these events occurs with the probability of p_i, $0 \leq p_i \leq 1$ and $\Sigma\, p_i = 1$.

The expected information content, or entropy, of a situation H (p) is the weighted sum of the individual events h (.), the weights being the respective probabilities (Xu et al., 2003):

$$H(p) = \Sigma\, p_i h(p_i) = \Sigma\, p_i ln\left(\frac{1}{p_i}\right) \tag{7.2}$$

This formula is a measure of the degree to which the probabilities of the various events are equal. It is obvious from equation (7.2) that the closer the p_i is to $\frac{1}{n}$, the smaller are the differences in probabilities and the greater is the entropy. A maximum is obtained when the probability of all events is equal; in that case, equation (7.2) becomes ln (n), as $p_i = \dfrac{1}{n}$.

T is a measure of the difference between the maximum and the expected information content of a situation, as follows (Xu et al., 2003):

$$T = \text{ln} \, (n) - H \, (p) \qquad (7.3)$$

Equation (7.3) can be written as:

$$T = \Sigma \, p_i \left[\text{ln}\,(n) - \text{ln}\left(\frac{1}{p_i}\right) \right] \qquad (7.4)$$

T, when applied to the income inequality measurement p_i, can be shown as $p_i = \dfrac{y_i}{\Sigma\, y_i}$, where y_i presents the income of the household i and $\Sigma \, y_i$ is the total income. Equation (7.4) can be written as (Xu et al., 2003):

$$T = \frac{1}{n} \Sigma \frac{y_i}{\mu} \, \text{ln} \left(\frac{y_i}{\mu}\right) \qquad (7.5)$$

In equation (7.5), μ represents the mean income. T is zero in the case of perfect equality, and higher values indicate high inequalities. This index has no upper limit. Thus, high index values represent high inequalities whereas low index values represent low inequalities (Xu et al., 2003).

MLD is another member of the family of entropy type of inequality measures. It is defined with equation (7.6) as follows:

$$\text{MLD} = \frac{1}{n} \Sigma \, \text{ln} \left(\frac{\mu}{y_i}\right) \qquad (7.6)$$

In equation (7.6), y_i represents the income of the household i, and μ is the mean income of all households. An index value of zero indicates perfect equality whereas higher values indicate higher inequalities. MLD has no upper limit like the T. Thus, MLD equals to zero in the case of perfect equality and high index values represent more inequality (Xu et al., 2003).

An alternative inequality index measure is the Atkinson index, which is one of the most popular welfare-based measures of inequality in the literature, and a commonly used measure of income inequality.

Atkinson index

The Atkinson index is an alternative measure of inequality found in the literature. Specifically, the distinctive feature of the Atkinson index is to examine the effect of inequalities in different areas of the income distribution enabling a more revealing quantitative assessment of qualitatively different inequities (Maio, 2007). Additionally, the Atkinson index makes assumptions on the underlying social welfare function and the relationship between transfers and changes in inequality (Xu et al., 2003). This index is interpreted as follows:

$$A = 1 - \left[\frac{1}{n} \Sigma \left(\frac{1 - HFK_i}{1 - HFK_0} \right)^{1-e} \right]^{1/(1-e)} \tag{7.7}$$

In this equation, HFK_i represents the financial contribution of household i and "e" is an inequality aversion parameter. Higher values of "e" indicate more inequality in healthcare system contributions. These relative differences vary as "e" increases. For example, when "e" increases from 0.40 to 0.55, more inequality is observed in the households' financial contribution at the tail of the distribution (Xu et al., 2003). The relative differences between countries vary as "e" increases. In countries where the increase is greater, there is more unfairness in the households' financial contribution at the tail of the distribution. Atkinson's index value also reflects the degree of concern given by higher values of the coefficient e (Xu et al., 2003).

Atkinson is one of the flexible index measures to examine the degree of inequality. It is also an alternative sensitivity measure to traditional inequality indices, such as the Gini index. Notably, several studies exist in the literature regarding the comparison of inequality indices. One of these studies conducted by Atems and Shand (2018) empirically examined the relationship between entrepreneurship and income inequality by using traditional inequality indices, such as Gini index and Atkinson index. It has been observed that Atkinson is a useful alternative to the Gini index (Atems and Shand, 2018).

Measurement of progressivity of distribution of OOP health expenditure

Progressivity analysis is a common way of understanding the distributive pattern of OOP health expenditures. This analysis helps to understand the degree of burden of OOP health expenditures considering the differences in the income level of households. A more illuminative approach to assessing the progressivity of healthcare financing systems is to employ progressivity indices (Wagstaff and van Doorslaer, 1992). Kakwani is a commonly used progressivity index measure (Kakwani, 1977). The following section gives more detailed information on Kakwani index measurement.

Kakwani index

The Kakwani index is a well-known indicator of progressivity. This approach measures the degree of progressivity. The Kakwani index is twice the area between Lorenz and concentration curves (Kakwani, 1977; Wagstaff and van Doorslaer, 1992).

The relative position of the Lorenz and concentration curves is the traditional method of examining departures from proportionality and identifying their location in the "ability to pay" distribution. The Kakwani index value (π_K) ranges from –2 to +1. Negative index values represent regressivity whereas positive index values represent progressivity (van de Poel et al., 2007). The resulting Kakwani index is twice the area between the Lorenz and concentration curves. The formulation of the Kakwani index is represented as the difference between concentration (C) and Gini (G) indices. G is a traditional measure of inequality of a distribution. It is defined as a value between 0 and 1, and the numerator is the area between the Lorenz curve and the line of equality (Wagstaff et al., 1989). Thus, the Kakwani index is the difference between these two indices, as follows:

$$\pi_K = C - G \qquad\qquad (7.8)$$

The Kakwani index provides an aggregate picture of tax progressivity and income distribution. This information is essential for applied welfare analysis (Ataguba, 2016). The bounds of the Kakwani index are dependent on the degree of pretax income inequality and ranges from –(1+GX) to (1–GX). Thus, these bounds point out the lowest regressivity and highest progressivity. The value of zero represents proportionality (Arcarons and Calonge, 2015). Therefore, different implications for the indices can be used according to the income distribution changes over time (Formby et al., 1981).

Nonetheless, incorporating curve approaches into the index analysis is the typical way of measuring inequalities. Obviously, one of the constraints of using multiple inequity indices is that two indices will represent different scores because they will give different weights to different parts of the distribution of interested inequity measure. Thus, it is possible to observe two different index scores applied in the same data. To overcome this limitation, the combination of index and curve approaches is essential in providing a more rational decision-making about the distributive pattern of OOP health expenditures (O'Donnell et al., 2008; Wagstaff et al., 1989; Wagstaff et al., 2011). The next section gives a very brief overview of Lorenz and concentration curves to inspect where they cross on the distribution.

Curve approaches

Lorenz curve

Curve approaches are complementary tools used to visualize the level of inequality in the distribution of healthcare services. The Lorenz curve is the traditional approach of detecting departures from proportionality and identifying their location in the "ability to pay" distribution (Maio, 2007).

In other words, Lorenz-based analysis is an established way of detecting departures from proportionality and examining their location in the ability to pay distribution. Lorenz curve has been widely used in public health, medical research, human service industry, and education. Social welfare analysis is the frequent application area of research of Lorenz curve (Luo and Qin, 2019).

The Lorenz curve indicates the area below the 45-degree line of equality because the lower-income groups in the income distribution earn less than their equal shares. The amount by which the Lorenz curve leaves the 45-degree line of equality is a measure of income inequality. Gini coefficient is the specific index measure of the area between the line of equality and Lorenz curve (Kakwani, 1977). The degree of departure of the concentration curve from the Lorenz curve in the downward direction indicates a more progressive OOP pattern (Maio, 2007).

Even though Lorenz-based analysis is one of the conventional methods of examining the degree of progressivity, its inability to provide a measure of the degree of progressivity is a limitation. As such, it is not possible to make comparisons across time and countries regarding the level of inequalities in healthcare (Lambert, 1993). The relative position of Lorenz and concentration curves is useful for equality analysis of the distribution of health expenditures.

Concentration curve

The concentration curve plots the cumulative percentage of the health sector variable (y-axis) against the cumulative percentage of the population ranked by living standards, beginning with the poorest and ending with the richest (x-axis) (Wagstaff and van Doorslaer, 1992).

In other words, the concentration curve plots the shares of the health sector variable against the share of the living standards variable. If everyone, irrespective of their living standard, has the same amount of the health variable or income and the same value of health or income variable, then the concentration curve will be a 45-degree line running from the bottom left-hand corner to the top right-hand corner – known as the line of equality. Contrarily, when the health sector variable takes higher (lower) values among poorer people, the concentration curve will lie above (below) line of equality. The farther the curve is above the line of equality, the more concentrated the health variable is among the vulnerable people (Wagstaff et al., 2011). The difference between the Lorenz curve and the concentration curve depends on what is being used as a ranking variable. The concentration curve represents the relationship between the variable for health and the variable for rank of the living standards; it does not represent the variable for variation in living standards itself (Wagstaff et al., 2011).

Visualization of Lorenz and concentration curves

Lorenz and concentration curves are visualized in Figure 7.1. A graphical representation of Lorenz and concentration curves show that on the horizontal axis, the population is classified and ranked according to income, from the lowest to the highest group. The vertical axis shows the total proportion of income within the community increasing in each group. Because the concentration curve lies at the bottom of the Lorenz curve, evidently the burden of income stands on the shoulders of wealthy households. In other words, the positions of Lorenz and concentration curves indicate a progressive pattern for the distribution of income (Wagstaff et al., 1989; Wagstaff and van Doorslaer, 1992).

Therefore, the visual representations of the Lorenz and concentration curves make it easy to determine regressivity or progressivity. However, the Gini coefficient is a specific measure to calculate the area between the Lorenz

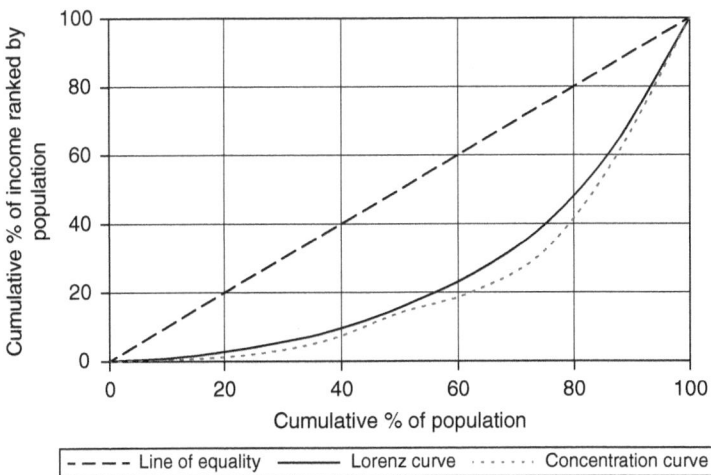

Figure 7.1 Lorenz and concentration curves.

Source: Adapted from Wagstaff and van Doorslaer (1992)

and concentration curve. Hence, the Gini index enables us to measure the area between Lorenz and concentration curves.

References

Arcarons J, Calonge S. (2015) Inference tests for tax progressivity and income redistribution: The Suits approach. *The Journal of Economic Inequality* 13(2):207–223.

Aronson JR. Johnson P, Lambert PJ. (1994) Redistributive effect and unequal income tax treatment. *The Economic Journal* 104(423):262–270.

Ataguba JE. (2016) Assessing equitable health financing for universal health coverage: A case study of South Africa. *Applied Economics* 48(35):3293–3306.

Atems B, Shand G. (2018) An empirical analysis of the relationship between entrepreneurship and income inequality. *Small Business Economics* 51(4):905–922.

Binagwaho, A., Nutt, C.T., Mutabazi V, Karema C, Nsanzimana S, Gasana M., Drobac PC, et al. (2013) Shared learning in an interconnected world: Innovations to advance global health equity. *Global Health* 9(37). https://doi.org/10.1186/1744-8603-9-37.

Cylus J, Roubal T, Ong P, Barber S. (2019) Sustainable Health Financing with an Ageing Population. www.euro.who.int/__data/assets/pdf_file/0008/411110/Sustainable_health_financing_with_an_ageing_population.pdf?ua=1. Accessed on: 1.3.2020.

Erreygers G, Clarke P, van Ourti T. (2012) "Mirror, mirror, on the wall, who is this land is the fairest of all?": Distributional sensitivity in the measurement of socioeconomic inequality of health. *Journal of Health Economics* 31(1):257–270.

Formby JP, Seaks TG, Smith WJ. (1981) A comparison of two new measures of tax progressivity. *The Economic Journal* 91(364):1015–1019.

Kakwani NC. (1977) Measurement of tax progressivity: An international comparison. *The Economic Journal* 87(345):71–80.

Lambert PJ. (1993). *The Distribution and Redistribution of Income: A Mathematical Analysis*. Second Edition. Manchester University Press: Manchester, UK.

Luo S, Qin G. (2019) Jackknife empirical likelihood-based inferences for Lorenz curve with kernel smoothing. Communications in Statistics–Theory and Methods 48(3):559–582.

Maio FGD. (2007). Income inequality measures. *Journal of Epidemiology & Community Health* 61(10):849–852.

O'Donnell O, van Doorslaer E, Wagstaff A, Lindelow M. (2008). *Analyzing Health Equity Using Household Survey Data: A Guide to Techniques and Their Implementation*. The World Bank: Washington, D.C.; 83–114.

van de Poel E, Hosseinpoor AR, Jehu-Appiah C, Vega J, Speybroeck N. (2007) Malnutrition and the disproportional burden on the poor: The case of Ghana. *International Journal for Equity in Health* 6(21):1–12.

Wagstaff A, van Doorslaer E, Paci P. (1989) Equity in the finance and delivery of health care: Some tentative cross-country comparisons. *Oxford Review of Economic Policy* 5(1):89–112.

Wagstaff A, van Doorslaer E. (1994) Measuring inequalities in health in the presence of multiple-category morbidity indicators. *Health Economics* 3(4):281–291.

Wagstaff A, Bilger M, Sajaia Z, Lokshin M. (2011) *Health equity and financial protection*. Streamlined Analysis with ADePT Software. The World Bank.

Wagstaff A, van Doorslaer E. (1992). Equity in the finance of health care: Some international comparisons. *Journal of Health Economics* 11(4):361–387.

Wagstaff A. (2000) Socioeconomic inequalities in child mortality: Comparisons across nine developing countries. *Bulletin of the World Health Organization* 78(1):19–29.

World Health Organization (WHO). (2010). Health systems financing: The path to universal coverage. World Health Report 2010: Geneva, Switzerland.

World Health Organization (WHO). (2013) Closing the Health Equity Gap: Policy Options and Opportunities for Action. Publications of the World Health Organization: Geneva, Switzerland. https://apps.who.int/iris/bitstream/handle/10665/78335/9789241505178_eng.pdf. Accessed on: 27.2.2020.

Xu K, Klavus J, Aguilar-Rivera AM, Carrin G, Zaramdini R, Murray CJL. (2003) *Summary measures of the distribution of household financial contributions to health*. Chapter 40, 543–555.

Chapter 8

Equity in pharmaceutical expenditures under health reform in Turkey

In Turkey, health reform environment affects out-of-pocket (OOP) health expenditure patterns of individuals (Yardım et al., 2014). Additionally, pharmaceutical expenditures constitute a significant part of OOP health expenditures. Therefore, pharmaceutical expenditure makes up a large share of total health expenditures in Turkey (Dorlach, 2016).

This book chapter concentrates on the distribution of the burden of pharmaceutical expenses in Turkey. Before analyzing the distributive pattern of pharmaceutical expenditures on households, an overview of the increasing level of OOP health expenditures is presented and internationally compared. After that, total pharmaceutical consumption in Turkey is monitored over the years, and lastly, Turkey's position in the global pharmaceutical market is examined and compared with other countries. Subsequently, index and curve approaches are used together for equity analysis of the distribution of pharmaceutical expenses in Turkey.

An overview of the level of OOP health expenditures and international comparison

In Turkey, the share of OOP health expenditure as a share of the total expenditure (%) over the years shows a fluctuating trend (see Figure 8.1). Notably, an apparent decline is observed for the year 2009. The numeric value of percentages started to decline after 2007 (MoH, 2015).

The declining trend of percentages is attributable to the reorganization in the health insurance market and more inclusive health policies. In other words, creating inclusive policies, establishing a general health insurance system, and providing more benefits to vulnerable groups are part of the cost–control mechanism. This mechanism will enable health policymakers in developing countries to efficiently use healthcare resources (Atun et al., 2016).

In Turkey, the degree of OOP current health expenditure as a share of total current health expenditure (%) has a low trend compared with developed Organization for Economic Co-operation and Development (OECD) 35 countries (MoH, 2015). Figure 8.2 shows the international comparison of

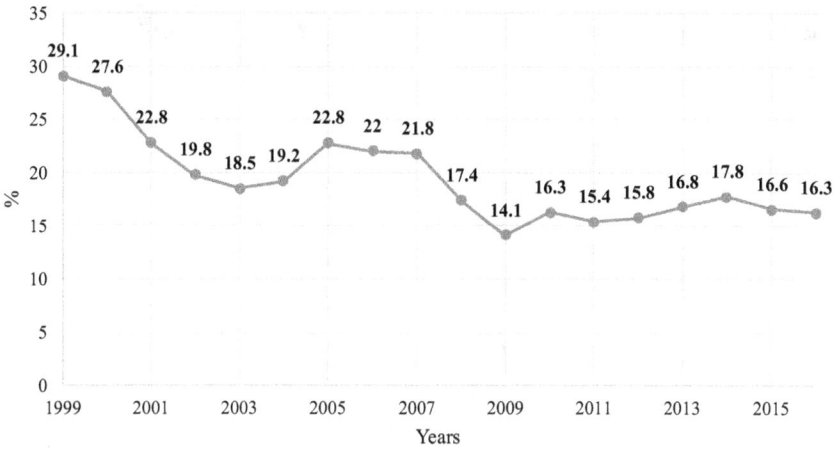

Figure 8.1 OOP health expenditure as a share of total health expenditure by years (%), Turkey.

Source: Turkish Ministry of Health Statistics Year Book (2015).

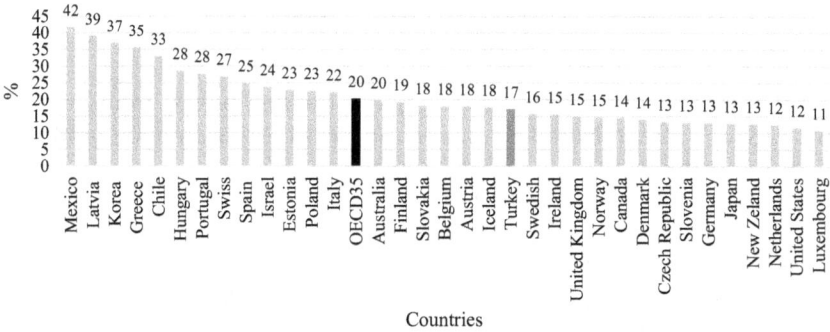

Figure 8.2 International comparison of OOP current health expenditure as a share of current health expenditure (%), 2014.

Source: Turkish Ministry of Health (MoH) Statistics Year Book 2015.

OOP current health expenditure as a share of total current health expenditure (%) for the year 2014. Turkey (16.5%) is below the OECD 35 countries average (20.3%).

Consumption of drugs (million boxes) and international comparison

Expenditure for pharmaceutical products and drugs constitute a significant part of OOP health expenditures. In Turkey, there is an increasing

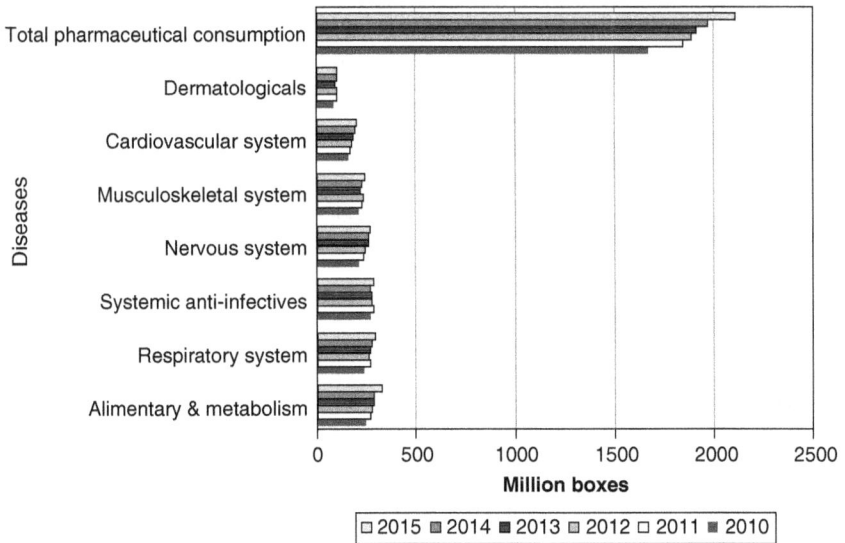

Figure 8.3 Consumption of drugs by years (million boxes), Turkey.

Source: Turkish Ministry of Health (MoH) Statistics Year Book 2015.

trend in total pharmaceutical consumption (million boxes) from 2010 to 2015 (MoH, 2015). Notably, total pharmaceutical consumption gradually increased between 2010 and 2015 (see Figure 8.3).

In addition, high consumption of drugs (million boxes) is consistent with current disease trends in Turkey. Consumption of million boxes of drugs as systemic anti-infectives and for treatment of diseases of alimentary canal and metabolism, respiratory system, nervous system, musculoskeletal system, cardiovascular system, and dermatological diseases has been high between 2010 and 2015 (MoH, 2015). Consistent with this information, low back disorders, which is one of the significant diseases, has been increasingly noted in individuals who are 15 years and above or the elderly in the year 2014 in Turkey. Total percentage of low back disorders (lumbago, back hernia, and other back defects) is 33%; neck disorders (neck pain, neck hernia, and other neck defects) is 21.3%; high blood pressure (hypertension) is 16.1%; and allergies, such as rhinitis, eye inflammation, dermatitis, food allergy, etc., are 12.1% (TurkStat, 2005–2015).

Growth potential of pharmaceutical market and international comparison

Turkey's pharmaceutical market has immense growth potential, and it is one of the pharmerging markets. The pharmaceutical market has

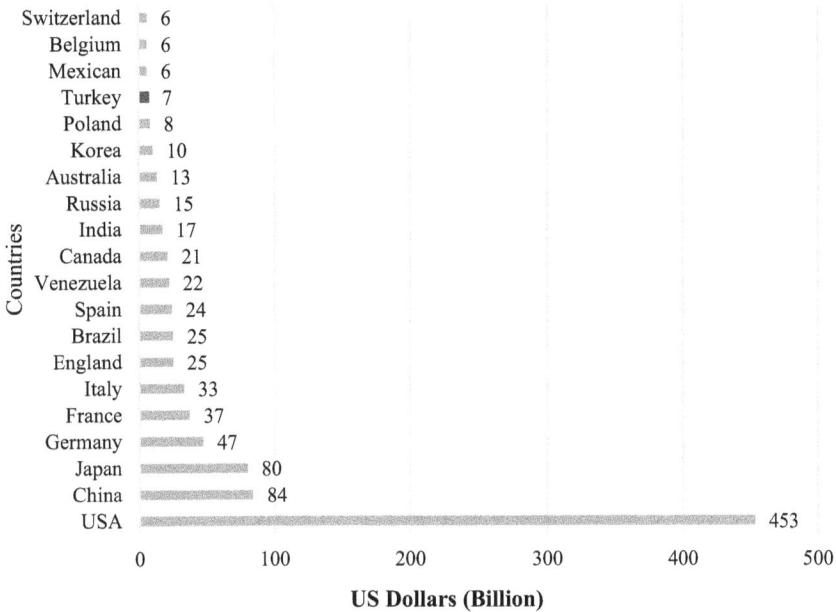

Figure 8.4 Worlds pharmaceutical market.

Source: Pharmaceutical Manufacturers Association of Turkey (IEIS) (2017).

achieved 1.10 trillion dollars for the year 2017 (IEIS, 2017). Turkey has tremendous pharmaceutical market growth potential and is one of the pharmerging countries that is 17th in the global pharmaceutical market (see Figure 8.4).

The pharmaceutical market growth potential, price policy in the pharmaceutical market, the share of the generic pharmaceutical market are significant indicators from a developmentalist perspective. When the price controls become stricter in developing countries, investment in domestic production becomes less likely. This price control is one of the main barriers of development in the pharmaceutical market and causes dependency of the pharmaceutical industry and dependency in the third world (Gereffi, 1983).

In Turkey, the percentage share of generic (value) in the total pharmaceutical market is high compared with other OECD countries (see Figure 8.5). Encouragement of the use of generic medicine is a strategy for the countries that have transition economies (King and Kanavos, 2002). The aim of the use of generic medicine and decrease in public pharmaceutical expenditure is achieved by financing the same medicine at lower prices. This aim can be considered as a strategy to protect vulnerable groups from the increasing level of pharmaceutical expenses (Dorlach, 2016).

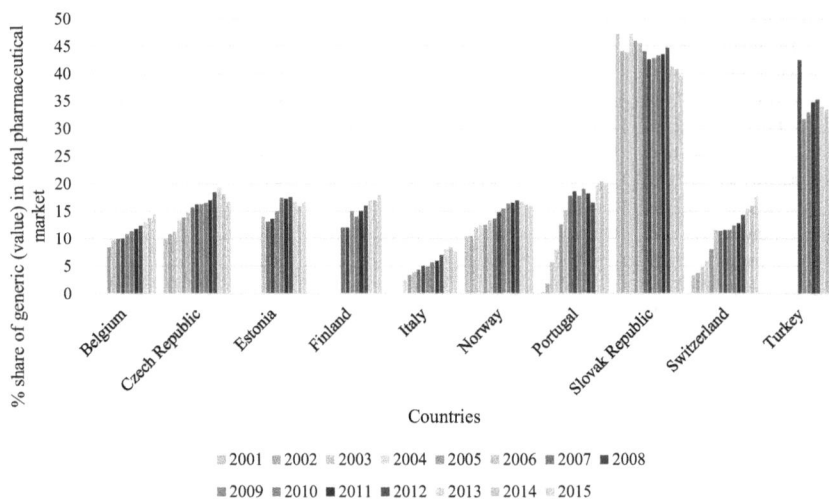

Figure 8.5 % share of generic value in total pharmaceutical market in Turkey and selected OECD countries.

Source: OECD. Stat Pharmaceutical Market. Generic Market 2001–2015.

Equity analysis of households' pharmaceutical expenditures in Turkey for the years 2005–2015

The increasing level of total pharmaceutical consumption from 2010 to 2015 necessitates to concentrating more on the level of pharmaceutical expenses. What is more crucial is to examine the distribution of pharmaceutical expenses in terms of equity perspective. To the best of our existing knowledge, there is a lack of knowledge about the distributive pattern of OOP pharmaceutical expenditures in Turkey.

To fill this void, in this book chapter, equity analysis of pharmaceutical expenditure has been examined by using the Household Budget Survey (HBS) data gathered from Turkish Statistical Institute (TurkStat) for the years 2005–2015.

In Turkey, HBS is a national survey, which mainly focuses on consumption expenditure. Household size and type, income, and expenditure groups are considered in the survey. Data are collected from a representative stratified clustered sample of households. The HBS was conducted between January 1 and December 31, including face-to-face interviews (TurkStat, 2005–2015).

The expenses of individuals were recorded in diaries by interviewers during the interview. The types of expenditures considered in the survey were food and nonalcoholic beverages, clothing, water, housing, and electricity. Health expenditures included the different functions of health services, such as pharmaceutical expenses, medical products, and out- and inpatient services (TurkStat, 2005–2015).

Sampling weights are provided from data files that are applied to the data of each year to generate nationally representative results. Prices were deflated using the consumer price index (CPI) for pharmaceutical products. The year 2005 was used as a base year for deflation. Turkish lira values were converted into 2005 prices using the CPI levels for monthly expenditure.

Descriptive statistics of total households, households that reported pharmaceutical expenses and CPI values for pharmaceutical products are presented in Table 8.1. It is noted that the percentage of households reporting pharmaceutical expenditures has increased over the years. (Note: the total number of households in the survey has increased as well.) In 2013, among surveyed households, a high percentage of households (60%) reported making a pharmaceutical expenditure.

Table 8.1 presents CPI values specific for pharmaceutical products between 2005 and 2015. These deflated values are used to analyze and compare pharmaceutical expenditures for the years 2005–2015.

Moreover, the percentage of households that reported pharmaceutical expenditure among the total number of households in the survey is presented in Table 8.1. It is observed that the percentage of households that reported pharmaceutical expenditures is more than 40%, indicating that a high percentage of households reported expenditure for pharmaceutical products. Despite small fluctuations, the percentage (%) of households reporting pharmaceutical expenditures increased from 2005 to 2013, before returning in 2015 to (almost) its starting level.

Changes in the percentage of households that reported pharmaceutical expenditures can be explained by structural changes and strong state regulations. In Turkey, after passage of the Act of 2006, and the Social Security and National Health Insurance Act of 2006 (amended in 2008), a single-payer system was established to enable all insured citizens equal access to healthcare services (Wendt et al., 2013). Before 2006, the level of healthcare coverage and changes in the quality of care among beneficiaries of the health insurance system were based on employment status (Akdağ, 2011). Health reform unified the different health insurance plans under the Social Security Institution (SSI), and harmonizing benefits and reimbursement rules. In addition, the Green Card project provided uninsured people with access to doctors and hospitals within the social security system; however, it did not cover pharmaceuticals. These structural changes are pioneering examples of inclusive policies and poverty alleviation strategies in healthcare (Akdag 2011; Agartan 2008; Yılmaz 2013). Under these regulations, the total public coverage rate increased from 67.2% in 2005 to 98.4% in 2015 (OECD 2017). In addition to the unification of health insurance system, important reforms in primary care with the establishment of a family medicine system enabled health services to become more accessible (Hone et al., 2017). Specifically, the total number of per capita visits to a physician in healthcare facilities increased from 3.1% in 2002 to 8.4% in 2015 (MoH, 2016).

In this regard, health financing reforms and primary care regulations incentivize using health services (Hone et al., 2017; Sozmen and Unal 2016), which in turn increases health expenditures (MoH, 2017). Supporting this statement: Turkish healthcare is characterized by high OOP payments, which on average comprised 22% of total healthcare costs from 2003 to 2008 (MoH, 2017). These regulations and changes in the health financing system may have encouraged healthcare consumers to use more health services and to spend more for these services than before. Because medicine is a costly area of healthcare in Turkey, households' pharmaceutical expenditures increased between 2010 and 2013 (MoH, 2015). Consistent with existing knowledge, the percentage of households reporting pharmaceutical expenditures increased slowly during the study years from 2003 to 2015 (see Table 8.1).

Strong state regulations to control pharmaceutical price increases may be another factor behind an increase in percentage of households that reported pharmaceutical expenditures. During the global economic crisis, Turkey implemented a strict pharmaceutical price policy as a part of the government's fiscal discipline (Vural 2015). This was supported by generic substitution of original drugs and the public financing of pharmaceutical expenditure (Dorlach, 2016). In the light of aforementioned strategies, the percentage of households reporting pharmaceutical expenditures slowly increased from 2005 to 2012, and then increased in 2013, the year that unification of the health insurance system was finalized. This percentage decreased in 2014, almost returning to its starting level in 2015, under continuing strict price control strategies to protect vulnerable groups (see Table 8.1).

We begin with descriptive statistics for pharmaceutical expenses of households and then examine a variety of index and curve approaches to examine the level of equity in terms of distribution of pharmaceutical expenses for the years 2005–2015.

First, mean monthly expenses for pharmaceutical products for the years 2005–2015 are presented in Figure 8.6. All price values are deflated, and an increasing trend is observed for mean monthly expenditures for pharmaceutical products over the study years.

All price values are deflated by using 2005 as a base year.

Descriptive statistics for pharmaceutical expenses of households for the years 2005–2015 are presented in detail in Table 8.2. Mean and median values of expenditure for pharmaceutical products and annual income are shown by using deflated values. CPI was used to calculate constant Turkish liras over the base year of 2005. Mean and median values of expenditure for pharmaceutical products show an increasing trend over the years. Table 8.2 also presents descriptive statistics for mean annual household income. It is

Table 8.1 Total number of households, households that reported pharmaceutical expenditure, and CPI values for pharmaceutical expenditures

Variables	Years										
	2005	2006	2007	2008	2009	2010	2011	2012	2013	2014	2015
Total number of households in the survey	8,559	8,558	8,548	8,549	10,046	10,082	9,918	9,987	10,060	10,122	11,491
Percentage of household's reported pharmaceutical expenditure	44%	46%	44%	47%	53%	53%	53%	52%	60%	53%	45%
CPI values*	84.93	88.02	83.90	87.81	93.10	92.15	89.91	91.69	93.33	98.88	106.43
Index deflate numbers	1	1.03	0.98	1.03	1.09	1.08	1.05	1.07	1.09	1.16	1.25

Source: TurkStat HBS for the years 2005–2015.

Note:
*CPI values for pharmaceutical products. To compare consumption internationally, in 2005, 1.34 Turkish liras = 1 US dollars (average), (Central Bank of the Republic of Turkey-CBRT, www.tcmb.gov.tr/. Accessed on: 11.02.2019).

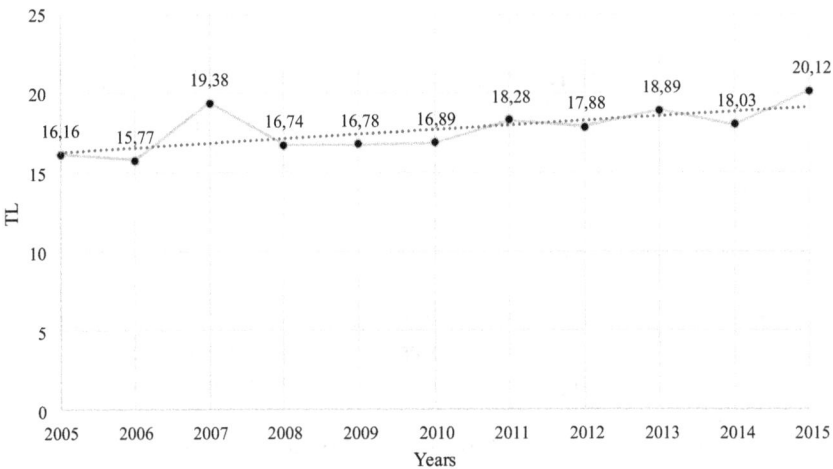

Figure 8.6 Mean monthly expenses for pharmaceutical products (TL), 2005–2015.

Source: TurkStat HBS for the years 2005–2015.

observed that there exists a general increasing trend for mean and median values of households' annual income from 2005 to 2015.

In Turkey, the increase in annual household income is consistent with general economic growth (Pamuk, 2019). Turkey's economic growth between 2002 and 2007 created a fiscal environment that supported financial protection strategies in healthcare (Pamuk, 2007). This growth was defined as "higher quality" because it depended on investments, innovation, and technology. Economic growth continued after 2007, but this growth was of "lower quality" (Acemoglu and Ucer, 2015). The influence of economic growth on a household's income has been debated and is still widely discussed regarding income inequality. Some economists argue that economic growth increases income inequality, whereas others argue the opposite (Atilgan et al., 2017). The welfare effect of economic growth on income inequality is controversial in the literature; in the meantime, inequalities in Turkey persist (Ergul and Cakir, 2019). Under inclusive health policies and poverty alleviation strategies under Turkey's Health Transformation Program, established in 2003, household's OOP health-related expenditures continue to increased (Wendt et al., 2013). Table 8.2 illustrates the consistent increases in annual income and pharmaceutical expenditures. Because healthy individuals benefit more from income growth and its welfare effects, the relationship between income and health expenditures must continue to be monitored so as to enhance global health.

The results of inequality index measures 2005–2015

In this case, values of inequality index measures are calculated using the "Inequality and Concentration Indices and Curves-IC2" package in R program. "IC2" allows the calculation of inequality and concentration index scores. Moreover, it enables understanding of the degree of progressivity by using the Kakwani index (Plat, 2015).

The results of Gini, Theil, mean logarithmic deviation (MLD), Atkinson, and concentration index results according to the burden of expenditure for pharmaceutical products are presented in Figure 8.7 for the years 2005–2015. Notably, high inequality index scores point to high levels of inequalities.

In this case, index scores allowed the following interpretations: (i) The trend for equal distribution of expenditure for pharmaceutical products generally had a steady and high trend between the years 2005–2015. (ii) The Gini index scores are higher than 0.50 for all the study years, and a high increase is observed for the year 2014. (iii) It is observed that the Atkinson index values are sensitive to the change in epsilon (e) parameter. In other words, "e" is an inequality aversion parameter in the Atkinson index. In this study, high values for Atkinson are observed for e = 2 (>0.70) than e = 1.5 (>0.60); e = 1 (>0.40), e = 0.50 (>0.20), and e = 0.25 (>0.10) for all the study

Table 8.2 Descriptive statistics for pharmaceutical expenses of households for the period 2005–2015

Descriptive statistics	2005	2006	2007	2008	2009	2010	2011	2012	2013	2014	2015
	Pharma expend.	Pharma expend.	Pharma expend.	Pharma expend.	Pharma expend.	Pharma expend.	Pharma expend.	Pharma expend.	Pharma expend.	Pharma expend.	Pharma expend.
Mean*	16.16	15.77	19.38	16.74	16.78	16.89	18.28	17.88	18.89	18.03	20.12
Median*	7.50	7.76	8.56	8.48	8.80	8.85	9.52	9.34	9.29	8.79	10.24
SE	0.48	0.44	0.66	0.50	0.50	0.53	0.47	0.54	0.53	0.39	0.67
Descriptive statistics	Annual income	Annual income	Annual income	Annual income	Annual income	Annual income	Annual income	Annual income	Annual income	Annual income	Annual income
Mean*	14781.13	15719	15308.15	15880.98	15383.25	16111.71	16857.36	18133.65	17854.88	18627.58	17946.50
Median*	11560.50	12536.68	12300.89	12307.32	12303.23	12446.16	13160.72	13907.79	14104.12	14462.68	14046.83
SE	221.60	206.55	221.76	232.48	184.74	226.99	218.69	289.47	218.44	266.06	245.84

Notes:
Pharma exp.: Expenses for pharmaceutical products (Turkish liras).

*Mean and median values of price values are deflated by using 2005 as a base year. SE: Standard error; in 2005, 1.34 Turkish liras = 1 US dollars (30.12.2005), (Central Bank of the Republic of Turkey-CBRT, www.tcmb.gov.tr/. Accessed on: 15.2.2019).

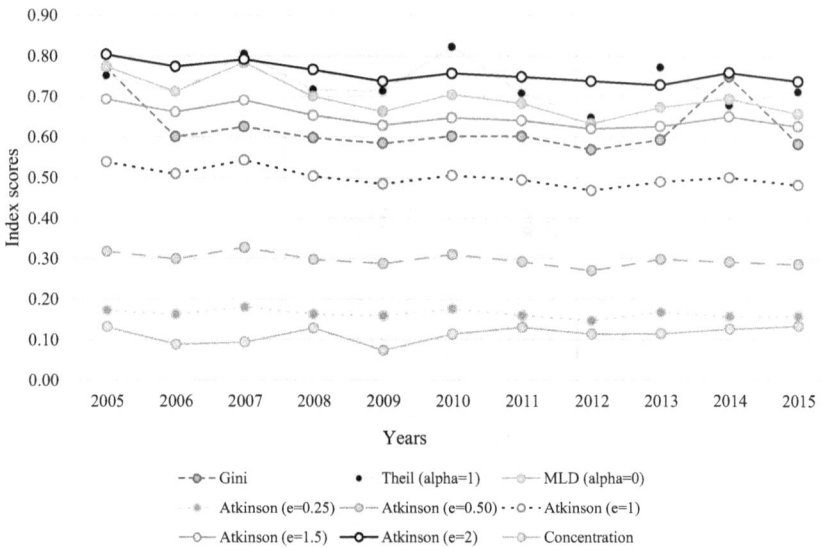

Figure 8.7 Results of inequality index scores, 2005–2015.

years. (iv) Entropy type of indices, which are Theil and MLD, show a steady and high trend for the study years.

Index scores for Theil and MLD are higher than 0.60 for all the study years. Index scores for concentration index are not interpreted here; it will be used to calculate and interpret the Kakwani index scores to examine the degree of progressivity of the distribution of expenditure for pharmaceutical products. Conclusively, inequality index scores indicate high levels of inequality in the distribution of expenditures for pharmaceuticals products for the years 2005–2015.

In this experiment, the Kruskal–Wallis (KW) variance analysis test was used to examine the statistical significance of the difference between inequality index scores. KW variance analysis test results indicate a statistically significant difference (X^2 = 90.18, p < 0.001) between inequality index scores for the years 2005–2015.

Progressivity analysis of the burden of pharmaceutical expenses, 2005–2015

The degree of progressivity of the burden of expenditure for pharmaceutical products is calculated using the Kakwani index scores. The Kakwani index is a well-known measure for progressivity analysis. It is calculated by finding the difference between the concentration index and the Gini index scores. To reiterate, the value of the Kakwani index ranges from –2 to 1. A negative index score indicates regressivity and verifies that the high amount of burden of pharmaceutical product expenses is placed on the shoulders of poor households (prorich). On the contrary, positive index scores point that high burden of pharmaceutical product expenses is placed on the shoulders of wealthy households (propoor) (Kakwani, 1977; Wagstaff et al., 1989)

In Turkey, the distribution of pharmaceutical product expenses shows a regressive trend (prorich) between 2005 and 2015. The Kakwani index values changed from –0.64 in 2005 to –0.45 in 2015 (see Figure 8.8). The regressive pattern of the distribution of the pharmaceutical product expenditure indicates the prowealth distribution of the financial burden of the pharmaceutical product expenses. It is critical to note that the Kakwani index became less regressive from 2005 to 2015 although the poor still bear the burden of OOP pharmaceutical expenses. Regressivity increased in 2014 and declined in 2015 given strict pharmaceutical price controls and public financing of pharmaceutical consumption. The lower regressivity from 2005 to 2015 evidences that the government's strict price control strategies protected vulnerable groups from the increasing burden of OOP pharmaceutical expenditures; however, index scores are still on the negative side. In other words, inequities have increased in Turkey in terms of the distribution of pharmaceutical expenditures from 2005 to 2015, and vulnerable groups are being adversely affected. Equity is the principal aim of a healthcare system, but there is considerable disagreement over the definitions and measurements of equity and its determinants (Liu et al., 2002). Pharmaceutical expenditures represent costly health maintenance in developing countries. In Turkey, poor populations have borne the burden of pharmaceutical expenditures from 2005 to 2015. It is clear that more inclusive policies are necessary to protect poor populations from increasing pharmaceutical expenditures. Regular monitoring of pharmaceutical and medical device prices, effective usage of fiscal space created by economic growth, overcoming rural–urban barriers to access healthcare services, improving health literacy, and promoting rational drug usage are advisable strategies to protect vulnerable groups from poverty immersion due to increasing pharmaceutical expenditures.

In light of this study, it can be stated that the burden of pharmaceutical expenses was placed on the shoulders of poor populations in Turkey for the years 2005–2015 – under the reformist environment in healthcare. To an egalitarian, an equitable healthcare financing system is the one where payments for healthcare are positively related to the ability to pay. In other words, the progressive burden of expenses is preferable than the regressive one (Wagstaff et al., 1989).

This interpretation is of relevance for developing countries because of financial resource constraints, income level differences, and high growth potential of the pharmaceutical market. Moreover, in Turkey, a high level of income differences exists in the population (Torul and Oztunalı, 2018). The results

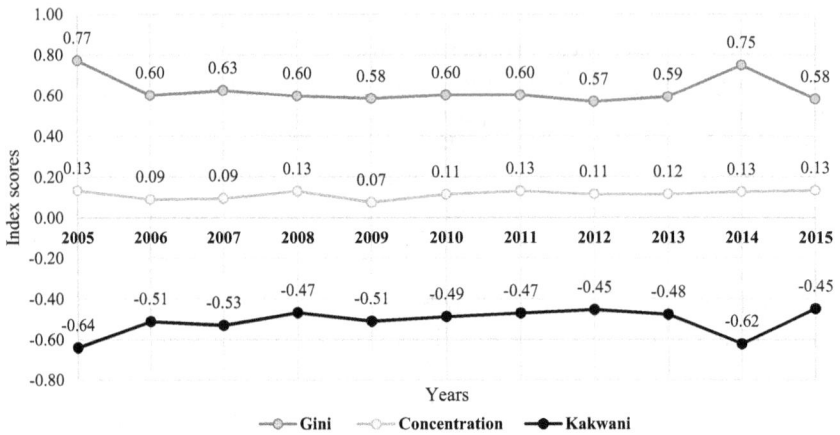

Figure 8.8 Kakwani index results for pharmaceutical product expenses for the years between 2005 and 2015.

of this case demonstrate significant results at the household level and verify that the burden of pharmaceutical expenses had a regressive pattern between 2005 and 2015, and vulnerable groups faced high risks with an increasing level of pharmaceutical expenditures. In Turkey, no statistics are available for the time before the Health Transformation Program was established; therefore, further research is necessary to verify the effects of health reform and to observe the changes in the regressive pattern of pharmaceutical expenses.

Progressivity analysis of burden of pharmaceutical product expenditures of households by using the Kakwani index scores for the years 2005–2015 clarifies a regressive (prorich) pattern in Turkey. However, a standard way of understanding the distributive pattern of expenditures in econometrics literature is to support index results with the curve approach because different indices are given different weights to different parts of the distribution of ability to pay.

In this regard, the curve approach provides supportive evidence to inspect where on the distribution the Lorenz and concentration curves cross. In light of these comments, the next section shows the Lorenz and concentration curves of the burden of pharmaceutical product expenditures.

Lorenz and concentration curves for 2005, 2010, and 2015

The visual representation of the degree of progressivity of the distribution of pharmaceutical expenses is presented in Figures 8.9, 8.10, and 8.11 for the years 2005, 2010, and 2015, respectively. The Excel program was used to illustrate the Lorenz and concentration curves and to determine the burden of the pharmaceutical expenditures on households.

2005

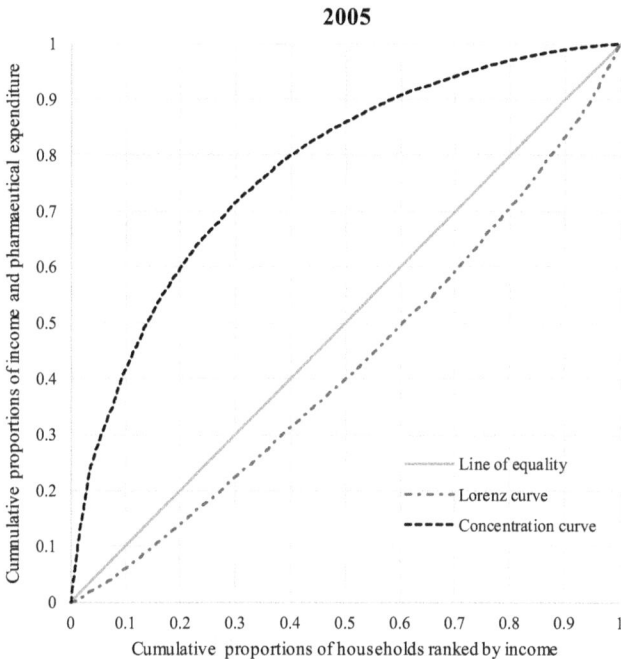

Figure 8.9 Lorenz and concentration curves for the year 2005.

Source: Author's own calculation by using TurkStat HBS for the year 2005.

Figure 8.9 presents the Lorenz and concentration curves for the year 2005. The concentration curve lies above the Lorenz curve indicating that the pharmaceutical expenditures are more regressively distributed than income. This regressive pattern is consistent with the Kakwani index results (2005; –0.64), which shows a prorich (inequity increasing) distribution of the financial burden of pharmaceutical expenditures for the year 2005. In other words, the distribution of the financial burden of pharmaceutical expenditures was on the shoulders of the poor households for the year 2005.

Figure 8.10 shows the relative position of the Lorenz and concentration curves for the year 2010. The distribution of expenditure for pharmaceutical products is still regressive implying that poorer households spent disproportionately more than their income on pharmaceutical products. The curve approach provides results consistent with the Kakwani index score which is –0.49 for the year 2010 and indicates a prorich distribution. Moreover, the distribution of pharmaceutical expenditures is less regressive for the year 2010 (KW = –0.49) compared with the year 2005 (KW = –0.64).

Figure 8.11 presents the Lorenz and concentration curves for the year 2015. The distribution of expenditure for pharmaceutical products has a regressive trend for the year 2015. In other words, there exists a prorich

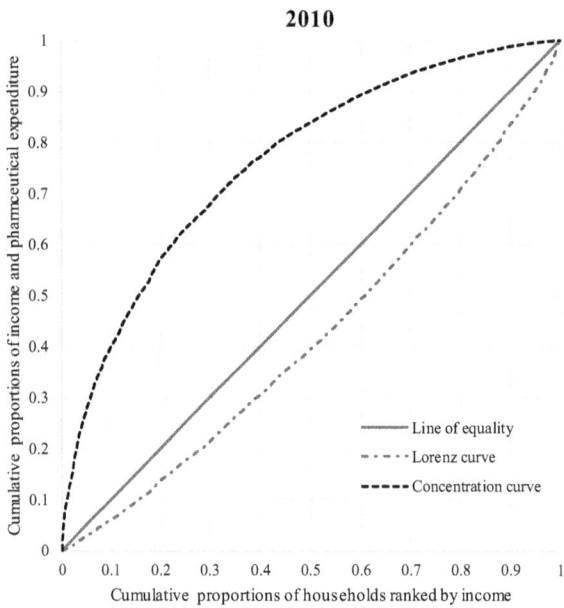

Figure 8.10 Lorenz and concentration curves for the year 2010.

Source: Author's own calculation by using TurkStat HBS for the year 2010.

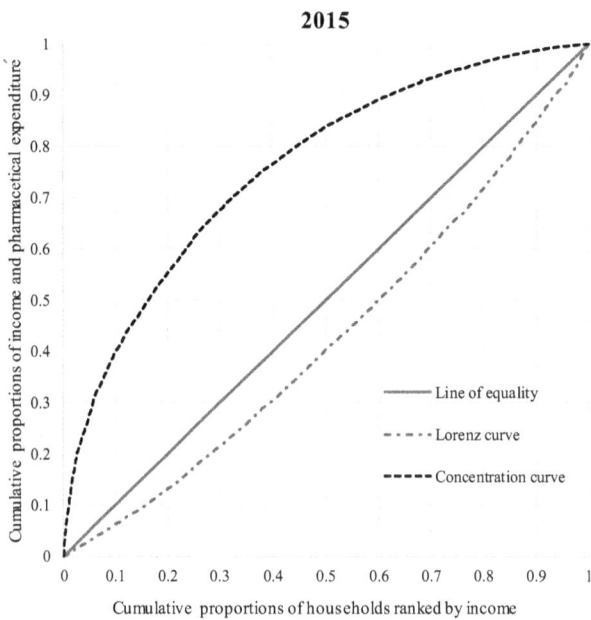

Figure 8.11 Lorenz and concentration curves for the year 2015.

Source: Author's own calculation by using TurkStat HBS for the year 2015.

(inequity increasing) distribution of the financial burden of pharmaceutical expenditures for the year 2015. The curve approach provides results consistent with the Kakwani index score, which is –0.45 for the year 2015. Additionally, the distribution of pharmaceutical expenditures is less regressive for the year 2015 (KW = –0.45) compared with the years 2010 (KW = –0.49) and 2005 (KW = –0.64).

The results of this case study show that in Turkey the distribution of pharmaceutical expenditures is regressive between 2005 and 2015. In other words, the burden of pharmaceutical expenses fell on the shoulders of poor households. These results clarify the existence of inequities for the study years.

The degree of regressivity is high for the year 2005; however, a less regressive trend is observed for the years 2010 and 2015. In other words, in Turkey pharmaceutical expenditure is regressive relative to the increase in the level of income under health reforms. In this case, equity analysis of the distribution of pharmaceutical expenditures contributes to a deeper understanding of the equity dynamics in pharmaceutical expenditure under inclusive health reforms in Turkey.

References

Acemoglu D, Ucer M. (2015) The ups and downs of Turkish growth, 2002–2015: Political dynamics, the european union and the institutional slide. NBER Working Paper 21608.

Agartan TI. (2008) Continuity and Change in Turkish Health Care System: The Challenge of Reform (A dissertation). Binghamton University, State University of New York: New York, USA.

Akdağ R. (2011) Türkiye sağlıkta dönüşüm programı değerlendirme raporu 2003–2011. [Turkey health transformation program assessment report 2003–2011] Ankara, Turkey: The Ministry of Health of the Republic of Turkey. https://sbu.saglik.gov.tr/Ekutuphane/Yayin/452. Accessed on: 8.5.2019.

Atilgan E, Kılıç D, Ertugrul HM. (2017) The dynamic relationship between health expenditure and economic growth: Is the health-led growth hypothesis valid for Turkey? *European Journal of Health Economics* 18(5):567–574.

Atun R, Chaumont C, Fitchett J, Haakenstad A, Kaberuka D. (2016). Poverty Alleviation and the Economic Benefits of Investing in Health. Ministerial Leadership Health in Program (ed). Harvard University.

Central Bank of the Republic of Turkey (CBRT). www.tcmb.gov.tr/ Accessed on: 15.2.2019.

Dorlach T. (2016) The AKP between populism and neoliberalism: Lessons from pharmaceutical policy. *New Perspectives on Turkey* 55:55–83.

Ergul IN, Cakir B. (2019) Inequality in Turkey: Looking beyond growth. https://arxiv.org/pdf/1910.11780.pdf. Accessed on: 8.9.2019.

Gereffi G. (1983) *The Pharmaceutical Industry and Dependency in the Third World.* Princeton University Press: Princeton, New Jersey, USA.

Hone T, Gurol-Urganci I, Millett C, Basara B, Akdag R, Atun R. (2017) Effect of primary health care reforms in Turkey on health service utilization and user satisfaction. *Health Policy and Planning* 32(1):57–67.

IEIS (2017). Turkish pharmaceutical market 2017. Pharmaceutical manufacturers association of Turkey. http://ieis.org.tr/ieis/en/sektorraporu2017/#page/2. Accessed on: 10.10.2019.

Kakwani NC. (1977) Measurement of tax progressivity: An international comparison. *The Economic Journal* 87(345):71–80.

King DR, Kanavos P. (2002) Encouraging the use of generic medicines: Implications for transition economies. *Croatian Medical Journal* 43(4):462–469.

Liu GG, Zhao Z, Cai R, Yamada T, Yamada T. (2002) Equity in health care access to: Assessing the urban health insurance reform in China. *Social Science & Medicine* 55(10):1779–1794.

Ministry of Health (MoH). (2017) Republic of Turkey, Ministry of Health Statistical Year Book (2017). https://dosyasb.saglik.gov.tr/Eklenti/31096,turkcesiydijiv1pdf.pdf?0. Accessed on: 10.10.2019.

Organization for Economic Co-operation and Development (OECD). (2017) Health at a Glance 2017-iLibrary; 2017. www.oecdilibrary.org/docserver/download/8117301e.pdf?expires=1521638527&id=id&accname=guest&checksum=A08F7E949C1F2536BE09B1ECB5F0D666. Accessed on: 10.03.2018

Organization for Economic Co-operation and Development (OECD). Stat Pharmaceutical Market. Generic Market 2001–2015. https://stats.oecd.org/Index.aspx?DataSetCode=SHA. Accessed on: 15.2.2019.

Pamuk S. (2007) Economic change in twentieth century Turkey: Is the glass more than half full? The American University of Paris. Working Paper. No. 41, pp. 1–32.

Pamuk S. (2019) Uneven centuries: Turkey's experience with economic development since 1820. The Economic History Review 72(4):1129–1151.

Plat D. (2015) Inequality and Concentration Indices and CurvesCurves-IC-2 Package https://cran.r-project.org/web/packages/IC2/IC2.pdf. Accessed on: 15.2.2019.

Sozmen K, Unal B. (2016) Explaining inequalities in health care utilization among Turkish adults: Findings from Health Survey 2008. *Health Policy* 120(1):100–110.

Torul O, Oztunalı O. (2018) On income and wealth inequality in Turkey. *Central Bank Review* 18(3):95–106.

Turkish Ministry of Health (MoH) Health Statistics Year Book. (2015). General Directorate of Health Research. Ankara. Turkey. https://dosyasb.saglik.gov.tr/Eklenti/6118,healthstatisticsyearbook2015pdf.pdf?0. Accessed on: 20.2.2019.

Turkish Ministry of Health Statistics Year Book. (MoH). (2016). https://dosyasb.saglik.gov.tr/Eklenti/13160,sy2016enpdf.pdf?0. Accessed on: 3.7.2019.

Turkish Statistical Institute (TurkStat) Turkey Health Survey 2005–2015. http://www.tuik.gov.tr/PreTablo.do?alt_id=1095. Accessed on: 5.7.2019.

Vural IE. (2015) Politics, reforms, and regulation of pharma prices and expenditures in Turkey over the 2000s. In Pharmaceutical Prices in the 21st Century, ed. Zaheer-Ud-Din Babar (pp. 267–295), Springer International: Cham, 2015, p. 289.

Wagstaff A, van Doorslaer E, Paci P. (1989) Equity in the finance and delivery of health care: Some tentative cross-country comparisons. *Oxford Review of Economic Policy* 5(1):89–112.

Wendt C, Agartan TI, Kaminska ME. (2013) Social health insurance without corporate actors: Changes in self-regulation in Germany, Poland and Turkey. *Social Science & Medicine* 86:88–95.

Yardım MS, Cilingiroglu N, Yardım N. (2014) Financial protection in health in Turkey: The effects of the Health Transformation Programme. *Health Policy and Planning* 29(2):177–192.

Yılmaz V. (2013) Changing origins of inequities in access to health care services in Turkey: From occupational status to income. *New Perspectives on Turkey* 48(48):55–77.

Chapter 9

Advice for health policymakers to consider equity in the distribution of pharmaceutical expenditures and pharmaceutical market design

Pharmaceutical expenses constitute a major part of health expenditures (Espin et al., 2018). An increase in pharmaceutical expenses threatens the financial sustainability of the health systems in developing countries such as Turkey. Turkey represents the developing part of the world, and its pharmaceutical market has significant growth potential. Therefore, this is one of the pharmerging countries (Civaner, 2012) and regulations in the pharmaceutical market have been one of the active policy areas of Justice and Development Party (Adalet ve Kalkınma Partisi – AKP) government since 2003, which is the when comprehensive Health Transformation Program (HTP) began (Dorlach, 2016).

In our case which is presented in Chapter 8, the level of equity in the distribution of pharmaceutical expenditures was examined, and the study results highlighted a regressive (prorich) pattern. This book chapter is based on a discussion of the question: "Are socially inclusive pharmaceutical reforms instrumental in nature and based on a rationale?,", and to answer this question better, specific advice for pharmaceutical policymakers are provided by trying to understand Turkey's cryptic and popular pharmaceutical policies under health reform atmosphere. Specific advice is provided for health policymakers regarding the necessity to consider the negative poverty effect of populist policies on the welfare state of individuals and the pharmaceutical market in Turkey.

Pharmaceutical market as an interactive policymaking area in healthcare

The pharmaceutical policies are undoubtedly multidimensional and consider issues related to public health, public expenditure, private sector dynamics, technological innovations, and industrial incentives (Aaserud et al., 2006; Tooole, 2012; Beletsi et al., 2018). Nonetheless, price levels and drug consumption patterns of individuals are other determinants of the level of pharmaceutical expenses (Ess et al., 2003).

High cost is one of the significant features of the pharmaceutical market in any country. However, the level of expenses differs according to the development level of the countries (Scherer, 2001). Cost containment is the primary motivation for European countries to control pharmaceutical expenditures. Health policymakers believe that high-price driven pharmaceutical expenditures are not sustainable and cause unfairness in pharmaceutical market design (Espin et al., 2018).

From a developmentalist perspective, price controls and regulations in the pharmaceutical market are determinants of growth of the pharmaceutical market. Thus, increasing the growth potential of the pharmaceutical market is essential to strengthen the economy of developing countries. If price controls become strict, then investments in domestic production become less likely (Gereffi, 1983; Dorlach, 2016).

Pharmaceutical market regulations and cost–control strategies must keep the broader picture in mind. Therefore, an evaluation through experimental and quasiexperimental studies is warranted for new policies (Ess et al., 2003).

The pharmaceutical policies are two-sided in nature. Although price controls play a significant role on the supply-side, continuous monitoring of individuals' drug consumption patterns plays a critical role in pharmaceutical market design (Griffiths et al., 2000). The crucial point of pharmaceutical policies from the demand-side is the lack of equity consideration. The absence of continuous monitoring of the level of equity in pharmaceutical expenditures and the shortage of planning about rational drug use are major shortcomings, especially in developing countries (Holloway and Henry, 2014). Developed country experiences show that if consumption of prescription drugs does not follow the need distribution, the consequence might be either overutilization, underutilizations, or horizontal inequity (Gundgaard, 2005). Therefore, pharmaceutical policies play a crucial role in healthcare equity.

On the other hand, health is a dynamic and uncertain policy environment, and health reforms are conceived to design the pharmaceutical market better. Inclusive policies and insurance market regulations are primary policy areas to protect vulnerable groups from the increasing level of pharmaceutical expenses (Ferrario and Kanavos, 2015).

Additionally, the pharmaceutical market is one of the interactive policy-making areas in healthcare. In other words, policymaking in the pharmaceutical market necessitates collaborative decision-making (Forster et al., 2014). Time and effort need to be invested in improving the quantity and quality of internationally comparable data on pharmaceutical expenditure that can provide the basis for analyzing the effect of different policies in various settings, which is crucial for low- and middle-income countries with scarce financial resources (Pejcic and Jakovljevic, 2017).

In this regard, continuous monitoring of the distributive pattern of the burden of pharmaceutical expenditures will enable policymakers to follow the level of pharmaceutical expenses regularly. Monitoring the level of equity in the pharmaceutical market is essential to ensure more sustainable finance of healthcare system (Pezzola and Sweet, 2016).

Progressivity analysis by using index and curve approaches are specific technical tools for health policy analysts. Health decisionmakers, technical advisors, and researchers from developed countries are more experienced regarding the use of these special techniques. They use these techniques for scientific and rational problem solving to address public health problems and improve health outcomes (O'Donnell et al., 2008). More data and knowledge sharing between developed and developing nations will provide significant benefits for regular monitoring of equity in the pharmaceutical market enabling cross-country comparisons and positively contributing to the growth of population health outcomes (Acosta et al., 2019).

Turkey's pharmaceutical policy reform and equity expenses

Turkey is one of the developing countries, and its pharmaceutical market has significant growth potential. Therefore, Turkey is called as one of the pharmerging markets. Turkey has experienced a substantial increase in the total pharmaceutical sales from USD 2.5 billion in 2002 to USD 8.0 billion in 2012 (SSI, 2019).

This increase is remarkable because the time period refers to the improved access to healthcare services after implementation of the Turkish HTP, which began in 2003 (Yılmaz et al., 2016). The magazine, Pharmaceutical Executive, announced that Turkey is one of the "pharmerging markets" and predicted annual growth of 11%–14% through 2013. The other pharmerging countries are Brazil, Russia, India, China, Mexico, and South Korea (Raymond and Chui, 2009).

Despite a low position in the pharmaceutical market, the pharmerging countries guarantee the sustainable development of the pharma industry because of their high speed of growth. Therefore, propagating the technological and scientific knowledge will help to enhance competitiveness in the market (Akkari et al., 2019).

The pharmaceutical market is private sector-driven and actors of the pharmaceutical sector modify their business activities to adapt themselves to current political trends in the pharmaceutical market (Reich, 1995). Therefore, understanding the current regulations in the pharmaceutical market coincides with the general policy of the government in any country. Turkey is a specific example to make interpretations on political economy and answer the question "why the Turkish government adopted populist rather than neoliberal policy solutions to solve high expenditure of the pharmaceutical industry?" (Dorlach, 2016).

Turkey's pharmaceutical policy reform

AKP's pharmaceutical policymaking can be understood by focusing on Turkey's pharmaceuticals policy reform, which began in September 2009 (Yılmaz et al., 2016). Turkey's economic growth is termed "high quality" between 2002 and 2007 based on the high level of productivity and transparent public management policies. However, this trend has changed, and the economic growth after 2007 has been termed "low quality" by economists (Acemoglu and Ucer, 2015).

High-quality economic growth created financial resources to improve the welfare distribution among the Turkish population (Acemoglu and Ucer, 2015). The distribution of resources is based on policymakers' choices, and AKP made its policymaking choice in favor of health market because healthcare is the major playground of AKP government and successfully reflected the voting behavior of individuals (Agartan, 2015). AKP's privilege in healthcare, as one of the former policy areas, makes it easy to understand the reason behind populist policies in pharmaceutical market regulations (Dorlach, 2016)

The global economic crisis had not directly affected Turkey's pharmaceutical market. However, post-2009, Turkey's pharmaceutical price policy was as a result of broader macroeconomic policy context, particularly related to the government's commitment to fiscal discipline. As a result of the broader macroeconomic policy context and the government's promise to maintain fiscal discipline, strict global budget defined AKP's pharmaceutical policy (Vural, 2015).

This policy was a solution to solve the increasing level of expenditures. However, during times of price increases, there exist two alternative solutions to solve this problem. First one is a neoliberal policy solution and increasing private share in the pharmaceutical market. The second one is strict price controls by increasing the share of the generic substation of prescribed original drugs. The second policy represents a populist health policy (Dorlach, 2016).

In Turkey, there exist two different approaches in pharmaceutical policymaking. One is represented by neoliberal-minded technocrats, who are the managers of economy and finance. They support using drugs rationally, increasing the role of the private sector, and improving the level of out-of-pocket health payments (Dorlach, 2016).

On the other hand, Prime Minister Erdogan is committed to a populist policy and opposed to reducing public financing of pharmaceutical consumption through classic neoliberal instruments. Health was one of the most popular policy areas of the AKP government, especially between 2002 and 2007 (Acemoglu and Ucer, 2015). Turkish policymakers chose the second alternative, which is a populist policy solution, thereby increasing the satisfaction of health services from 40% to 76% between 2003 and 2011 (MoH, 2015).

Erdogan proposed that reducing public financing of pharmaceuticals consumption could result in less electoral support because of the less access to public health services, especially for AKP's vulnerable supporters. Erdogan undoubtedly understood the high electoral cost of incorporating neoliberal market policies into the pharmaceutical market and strongly supported popular policies and strict market policy. Therefore, generic substitution of prescribed original drugs increased and Turkey became one of the pharmerging countries with a strong growth potential of the pharmaceutical market (Dorlach, 2016; Kockaya et al., 2017; Yılmaz et al., 2016). Under these policies, pharmaceutical products account for exorbitant spending on healthcare in Turkey, and the generic drug market has high growth potential (WHO, 2015). Public pharmaceutical expenses increased gradually during the period of health reforms: for the years 1994, 2002, and 2011, these expenditures were 5.734 million TL, 13.430 million TL, and 15.865 million TL, respectively (MoH, 2015). Moreover, according to projections of public pharmaceutical expenditures in the future, public pharmaceutical expenditures are expected to reach 38.547 million TL in 2020 (Ministry of Finance, 2017).

The core element of the AKP's populist discourse centered on cost-containment strategies in the pharmaceutical sector as implemented by the HTP. The rhetoric of redistribution was adopted by the government to protect vulnerable groups (Acemoglu et al., 2013) through its pharmaceutical price policy. Over the years, this price policy for medicinal drugs has become one of the major areas in which the government attracts the interest of median voters and avoids any loss of electoral support because of increases in pharmaceutical prices. Thus, a strict price rule and expenditure controls are the main tenets of the AKP's populist pharmaceutical policies (Dorlach, 2016)

Between 2004 and 2008, the neoliberal reforms in healthcare were supplemented by pharmaceutical price guidelines and expenditure control policies. Before the reforms, the Ministry of Health (MoH) regulated the maximum market price of pharmaceuticals through a cost and control scheme, and the fragmented social security schemes previously mentioned had their own uncoordinated cost-containment measures (Vural, 2017). Two separate price-control mechanisms have been instituted through the HTP. The first, control over maximum market prices of pharmaceuticals, is regulated through the External Reference Pricing System, implemented by the MoH. Second, a set of supply-side expenditure control measures are applied by the SSI, which has emerged as a monopolistic public purchaser of health-related services and pharmaceuticals since the centralizations of healthcare (Vural, 2015).

Transformations in healthcare have generated new challenges for the pharmaceutical industry, and Turkey appears to have become the stage for neoliberal pharmaceutical reforms since 2009 (Dorlach, 2016; Vural, 2015;

2017). After 2009, the government increased stringency of its pharmaceutical pricing and control policies to reduce public expenditures and to stabilize the short-term, capital-led growth model (Vural, 2015). These policies compelled international pharmaceutical companies and foreign multinational pharmaceutical producers to prepare a report for Turkey's government in which they advised the relaxation of regulations of pharmaceutical pricing and reimbursement and asked for the renewed expansion of public pharmaceutical expenditures. However, because of the electoral costs of cutting health expenditures, the government has continued its strict price policy. In fact, during the later phases of its health reform program, the Turkish government was faced with a policy shift among electoral interests, business interests, and industrial strategy (Dorlach, 2016).

Surprisingly, despite the obvious increase in pharmaceutical expenditures, the quantum of pharmaceutical expenditure is reducing healthcare inequity. Furthermore, these expenditures constitute one of the primary facets of the AKP's populist rhetoric and strongly affect voter preferences (Dorlach, 2016). The increase in household pharmaceutical spending in Turkey has had unsatisfactory outcomes (Agartan, 2012, 2015). Thus, the redistributive effects of the government's populist pharmaceutical policies have become a field of intense research.

The effect of Turkey's pharmaceutical policy reform on equity in the burden of pharmaceutical expenses

In our case, the degree of equity in the burden of pharmaceutical expenses in Turkey shows a regressive trend between 2005 and 2015, which is the period that coincides with AKP's strong commitment to HTP.

In other words, redistributive politics and reorganizations of the health system are the central dynamics of health reform atmosphere (Atun et al., 2013). After 2009, strict price policy became one of the dominant tenets of AKP's pharmaceutical policy. Even though the primary motive of this policy was to protect the poor population from high pharmaceutical expenditures, our case results differ from that and show that the burden of pharmaceutical expenditures is on the shoulders of the vulnerable groups.

In other words, AKP's strong commitment to protecting the poor population from increasing pharmaceutical expenditures failed to guard financially weaker groups between 2005 and 2015. Notably, the level of regressivity is high for the year 2005 with the Kakwani index value of –0.65. However, 2005 refers to the period when AKP's strict price policy had not come into force. After 2005, the degree of regressivity started to decrease. The distribution of pharmaceutical expenses in Turkey shows a steady regressive trend after 2009 under strict pharmaceutical price regulations. In our case, it is observed that the distributive trend of expenditure for pharmaceutical products is regressive and the burden is on financially weaker population.

On the other hand, another reason for the Turkish government to maintain its strict price policy is the lack of powerful business interests in high prices among the staunch supporters of the AKP government. The supportive business community of AKP is called as "Anatolian capital." These consist of conservative business people who were not active in pharmaceutical production and had little interest in the level of medicine prices before the year 2009 (Dorlach, 2016).

Furthermore, there existed significant communication problems between 2009 and 2012 between the AKP government and the dominant foreign business community in the pharmaceutical market. However, the dominance of foreign ownership in the pharmaceutical market has changed after 2009 (Dorlach, 2016; Kumru and Top, 2018).

New companies that are representatives of "Anatolian capital" came into force and became one of Turkey's generic manufacturers and exporters. Under the effect of the strong growth potential of the pharmaceutical market in Turkey, "national pharmaceutical" was announced by Erdogan in 2013 (Dorlach, 2016). The reason behind this announcement was that despite the high profitability in the drug sector, there was a relative decline in local products (Akgul and Koprulu, 2017).

To sum up, commitment to strict pharmaceutical price policy, increasing growth potential of the pharmaceutical market, and generic drug use are signs that populist policies are dominant in AKP's pharmaceutical market and price regulations (Dorlach, 2016).

In other words, it is possible to interpret that the interests of lower-class voters shape AKP's pharmaceutical policymaking (Bugra and Keyder, 2006). Therefore, it can be interpreted that AKP can implement propoor and socially inclusive policies in the pharmaceutical market (Vural 2015; Dorlach 2016).

However, AKP's pharmaceutical policies need to be analyzed from the equity perspective, and it is necessary to examine the degree of progressivity of the distribution of pharmaceutical expenses.

Our case study fills this void by providing evidence that the distribution of pharmaceutical expenses was regressive and placed on the shoulders of the poor population between 2005 and 2015. Therefore, the "social face" of AKP regulations in the pharmaceutical market did not rationally support the health expenditures of Turkish households. In other words, pharmaceutical market control strategies are not instrumental.

Advice for Turkish health policymakers to consider equity in pharmaceutical market design and price controls

In this regard, several advice are provided to Turkish health policymakers to consider equity in pharmaceutical market design and price controls. Pharma industry is essential for the development of the health sector in developing countries like Turkey (Lichtenberg et al., 2017).

Therefore, continuous monitoring of the level of equity in pharmaceutical expenses is strongly advised to know if the inclusive policies reflect on households' expenditures (Gemmill et al., 2008). Moreover, price controls, continuous monitoring of the increase in households' pharmaceutical expenditures, development of sustainable high-price industrial policy strategies and strong communication channels with the pharma industry were the prior strategies to enhance the pharma market.

For developed European countries, the primary goal for pharmaceutical expenditure is cost containment. This goal is owing to the general belief among healthcare policymakers that pharmaceutical expenditure – driven by high prices – will be unsustainable unless further reforms are not achieved (Espin et al., 2018).

Moreover, developed European countries control prices with just a few control profits. The effects of price controls on the overall price differences have been ambiguous. Although prices tend to be lower in countries with fixed prices, price controls have created implicit incentives toward "me-too" products (Ess et al., 2003).

Turkish policymakers strongly support national drug production (Tengilimoglu et al., 2005). It is essential to know that political commitment to the industrial development of the domestic pharmaceutical sector generally implies more affordable regulation of pharmaceutical prices. If national regulators of a capitalist economy wish to increase investments in domestic production, they need to ensure that these investments are profitable. When price controls become stricter, the investments in domestic production become less likely (Lambrelli and O'Donnell, 2011; Kyle, 2007).

Strong growth potential of generic drug market necessitates specific policy advice for Turkish policymakers in the pharmaceutical market in the light of the regressive burden of pharmaceutical expenditures on households. Generic drugs play a prominent role in efficiently allocating financial resources for pharmaceutical medicines (Kumru and Top, 2018). Evidence from developed countries encourages the use of generic medicines. Price competition is useful and will improve efficiency in the pharmaceutical market. Therefore, developing countries must be adapt to developed country experiences and consider local conditions, rural–urban dynamics when regulating generic drug market (King and Kanavos, 2002).

Turkey is a specific example of a country with strong development potential of the generic drug market and strict price regulations (Kumru and Top, 2018; Vural-Eren 2015). Support of the growth of the generic drug market and price constraints together form "price-control" mechanisms in the pharmaceutical market. However, the literature shows that price control is ineffective in controlling drug expenditure and causes undesirable distributive effects (Atella, 2000).

On the other hand, pharmaceutical product consumers' welfare has a two-sided nature. The first side represents improving clinical benefits with the use of pharmaceutical products. The second side is related to the level of pharmaceutical product price and relative comparison of the levels of pharmaceutical market prices with income of individuals.

The need to put inclusive policies on a rational basis

Our case shows that the distribution of pharmaceutical expenditures shows a regressive trend between 2005 and 2015. The trend of regressivity is high for the years 2005 (KW = −0.64) and 2014 (KW = −0.62). The relative positions of Lorenz and concentration curves confirm prorich (inequity increasing) distribution of pharmaceutical product expenditures.

It is known that AKP's strict pharmaceutical price policy began in 2009 (Dorlach 2016; Vural, 2015). Inequity trend of distribution of pharmaceutical product expenses shows a relatively small level of the regressive trend between 2010 and 2013. Our case study provides exciting findings regarding this and verifies less regressive trend for the years 2010–2013 when AKP's strict pharmaceutical price-control strategy began and continued. Additionally, this period represents the time when AKP's socially inclusive policies existed in the health market. Improvement of insurance coverage, increment of health benefits for poor populations, and enhancement of accessibility of health services with strong primary health system make the health sector a star among the other policies of AKP government (Agartan 2015).

Our case also provides supportive information regarding the increased level of expenditure for pharmaceutical products between 2005 and 2015. A high level of pharmaceutical product expenditures was observed in 2007 compared with other years.

The results of this study show that inclusive and populist policies to control the increase in pharmaceutical expenses failed to have a rational basis. We found that the burden of household expenditure on healthcare is not equally distributed among different income groups. Households from the lowest income quintile pay a larger share of their income on pharmaceutical products compared with households in the highest income quintile.

Furthermore, strict price policy is the main feature of AKP's pharmaceutical policy. Under the strict price policies, poor population is placed at a disadvantage, and they spend disproportionately more than their income on pharmaceutical products (Vural-Eren 2015). Notably, increasing the health benefits and insurance coverage are incentivizing factors for health consumers to use more health services and spend more on healthcare (Anderson et al., 2010).

Therefore, it is possible to interpret that Turkish households spend more on pharmaceutical products under the effect of redistributive policies in the health market. Curiously, Turkish households are spending more on healthcare than before, but they continue to be satisfied with health services (Hone et al., 2017). High level of satisfaction of Turkish households from health reform implications, high popularity of health reforms among the other policies of AKP, and incorporation of welfare state outsiders into the system are the attractive objectives of policymakers with an electoral focus.

However, increasing awareness of the Turkish government regarding high level of pharmaceutical expenses brings on to the table the need to make new financial resource distribution decisions and choose between different policy options. Additionally, before 2009, AKP's strong supporters were not dominant in the pharmaceutical market and there existed a lack of communication with the foreign pharmaceutical market. Strict price control started in 2009 to control increasing pharmaceutical expenses and encourage national drug production (Dorlach, 2016).

However, our case shows that policy motivations of AKP government did not reflect the welfare distribution of households. Our interpretations are broadly in line with the existing knowledge and ascertain that the economic term "populism" refers to the policies of redistribution and this often causes negative financial consequences (Acemoglu et al., 2013).

Health policymakers need to consider that populist policies have negative poverty effect on welfare state of individuals

The effect of the global rise of populist policies on the level of welfare states of households has garnered the interest of researchers. Scholars suggest that populist policies have negative poverty effect on the welfare state of individuals. Unfair redistributive policies, unequal access to welfare benefits, and increased health inequalities are some of the negative effects of popular policies (Stuckler, 2017; Greer et al., 2017; Acemoglu et al., 2013; Rodrik, 2018).

Moreover, inclusive policies have resulted in a significant economic crisis that affected the poorer segments of the population (Dornbusch and Edwards, 1991). In this regard, existing knowledge supports our findings and emphasizes the regressive effect of strict pharmaceutical price policy of the AKP government (Acemoglu et al., 2013).

It is thought-provoking why politicians adopt such policies and receive support for it. The answer to this question lies in the existence of high levels of inequality and weak political institutions in these countries. Therefore, politicians continue their redistributive rhetoric, but they continue their policies to provide more benefits for the elite (Acemoglu et al., 2013).

To sum up, consistent with the existing literature, Turkey's inclusive policies harm rather than help much of the population in terms of distribution of pharmaceutical expenditures. Even though the median voters are suffering from redistributive policies, they continue to support AKP's health policies.

In this regard, it is highly advisable for health policymakers in Turkey to consider the poverty effect of pharmaceutical market price regulations. Focusing on income level differences and developing protective policies for poor populations are essential to ensure an equitable pharmaceutical market.

On the other hand, increased use of generic drugs is highly supported by the AKP government as a mechanism to control the increasing level of pharmaceutical expenses. Notably, the existence of the generic drug market is crucial for developing countries for the development of their pharmaceutical market (Moon et al., 2011).

Generic drug market design and the need for high-priced industrial policy strategy

The existence of the generic drug market is one of the cost–control strategies for OECD countries (OECD, 2017). Turkey is one of the pharmerging countries, and the generic market has a large share (Yilmaz, 2016). Besides the growth potential of the generic drug market, health policymakers in Turkey need to be aware of the dominant generic producers in the market. Moreover, the development of "national pharmaceutical" was supported by Erdogan since 2013. After 2009, some local generic producers closely associated to the AKP emerged in the pharmaceutical market (Dorlach, 2016).

Health policymakers need to provide equal benefits to the different producers to improve the quality and competitiveness and develop high-quality products for customers (Sirgy et al., 2011). Therefore, it is highly recommended that health policymakers provide equal opportunities for producers to build a sustainable pharmaceutical market. From a different perspective, despite encouraging the use of generic drugs in Turkey, there is limited knowledge regarding the perception and attitude of health professionals and consumers on generic drug use (Toklu et al., 2012).

Therefore, education programs are necessary to improve the knowledge of health professionals and health consumers to enhance the effectiveness of the generic drug market. One of the drawbacks of AKP's pharmaceutical policy is the absence of high-price industrial strategy (Dorlach 2016).

In other words, sustainability of the low-price policy in the pharmaceutical market, which is highly competitive, necessitates the development of strategies for high-price policy (Pérez-Casas et al., 2001). Pharmaceutical policy leaders need to overcome the problem of the absence of commitment to development in the pharmaceutical sector industry policy (Chen et al., 2019).

To conclude, new reforms to redesign the pharmaceutical market are necessary for the sustainability of the healthcare system in Turkey. In other words, providing additional benefits for the vulnerable groups is advisable for health policymakers to manage welfare dynamics in the country better. More attention should be paid to the protection of the vulnerable social groups (specifically, the poor) when implementing patient charges for pharmaceutical products.

Furthermore, opposing the informal payments is essential to improve equity in healthcare financing and avoid inequalities in accessing healthcare. Informal payments for health services is one of the problems of health sector in Turkey (Tatar et al., 2007). Education programs are advisable strategies to enlighten the physicians and consumers for enhancing their prescribing and purchasing attitudes, respectively. Moreover, Turkey has been criticized because of the lack of communication with the pharmaceutical industry (Dorlach, 2016). Advice is warranted regarding the need for real and logical industrial policy strategy for the pharmaceutical sector. High-price policy strategy development is strongly recommended.

Therefore, it is highly advisable to improve communication channels with pharmaceutical industry representatives. Finally, Turkey is undergoing new health reforms, including the construction of city hospitals. City hospitals are specific public–private partnership (PPP) management models in healthcare and popular in the UK. Turkey is the leader among the European countries regarding its high investment in PPP models (EPEC, 2017).

High levels of investment on PPP introduces debate on the effective management of public health resources (Barlow et al., 2013; Osei-Kyei and Chan, 2015; Top and Sungur, 2018). However, there is a lack of knowledge about the effect of this reorganizations process on the pharmaceutical market and the level of pharmaceutical prices (Croft, 2005; Laverty et al., 2012).

Future studies will examine the equity effect of current policy implementations on the pharmaceutical market. Overall, it is imperative to bear in mind that for achieving healthcare equality, a nonmarket financing scheme that treats healthcare as a human right is essential. However, the existence of developmental industrial policy strategies is necessary to improve the pharmaceutical market, which is especially critical from a developmentalist perspective. To conclude, continuous monitoring of the distributive pattern of pharmaceutical expenditures is essential to ensure equity and better distribution of resources in health services in Turkey.

References

Aaserud M, Austvoll-Dahlgren A, Kösters JP, Oxman AD, Ramsay C, Sturn H. (2006) Pharmaceutical policies: Effects of reference pricing, other pricing, and purchasing policies. Cochrane Systematic Review – Intervention. https://doi.org/10.1002/14651858.CD005979.

Acemoglu D, Egorov G, Sonin K. (2013) A political theory of populism. *The Quarterly Journal of Economics* 128(2):771–805.

Acemoglu D, Ucer M. (2015) The ups and downs of Turkish growth, 2002–2015: Political dynamics, the European Union and the institutional slide. NBER Working Paper No. 21608.

Acosta A, Vanegas EP, Rovira J, Godman B, Bochenek T. (2019) Medicine shortages: Gaps between countries and global perspectives. *Frontiers in Pharmacology* 10:1–21.

Agartan TI. (2012) Marketization and universalism: Crafting the right balance in the Turkish health care system. *Current Sociology* 60(4):456–471.

Agartan TI. (2015) Explaining large-scale policy change in the Turkish health care system: Ideas, institutions, and political actors. *Journal of Health Politics, Policy and Law* 40(5):971–999.

Akgul A, Koprulu OM. (2017) Turkish drug policies since 2000: A triangulated analysis of national and international dynamics. *International Journal of Law, Crime and Justice* 48:65–79.

Akkari ACS, Munhoz IP, Santos NMBF. (2019) USA, Europe and pharmerging countries: A panorama of pharmaceutical innovation. In: Mula J., Barbastefano R., Díaz-Madroñero M., Poler R. (eds) *New Global Perspectives on Industrial Engineering and Management*. Lecture Notes in Management and Industrial Engineering. Springer: Cham, Switzerland.

Anderson M, Dobkin C, Gross T. (2010) The effect of health insurance coverage on the use of medical services. NBER Working Paper Series. Working Paper 15823.

Atella V. (2000) Drug cost containment policies in Italy: Are they really effective in the long-run? The case of minimum reference price. *Health Policy* 50(3):197–218.

Atun R, Aydın S, Chakraborty S, Sümer S, Aran M, Gürol I, Nazlıoğlu S, Ozgülcü S, Aydoğan U, Ayar B, Dilmen U, Akdağ R. (2013) Universal health coverage in Turkey: Enhancement of equity. *The Lancet* 382(9886):65–99.

Barlow J, Roehrich J, Wright S. (2013) Europe sees mixed results from public-private partnerships for building and managing health care facilities and services. *Health Affairs* (Millwood) 32(1):146–154.

Beletsi A, Koutrafouri V, Karampli E, Pavi E. (2018) Comparing use of health technology assessment in pharmaceutical policy among earlier and more recent adopters in the European Union. Value in Health Regional Issues. 16:81–91.

Bugra A, Keyder C. (2006) The Turkish welfare regime in transformation. *Journal of European Social Policy* 16(3):211–228.

Chen X, Yang H, Wang X. (2019) Effects of price cap regulation on the pharmaceutical supply chain. *Journal of Business Research* 97:281–290.

Civaner M. (2012) Sale strategies of pharmaceutical companies in a "pharmerging" country: The problems will not improve if the gaps remain. *Health Policy* 106(3):225–232.

Croft SL. (2005) Public-private partnership: From there to here. *Transactions of the Royal Society of Tropical Medicine and Hygiene* 99(1):9–14.

Dorlach T. (2016) The AKP between populism and neoliberalism: Lessons from pharmaceutical policy. *New Perspectives on Turkey* 55:55–83.

Dornbusch R, Edwards S. (1991) The Macroeconomics of Populism in Latin America. Retrieved from: www.nber.org/books/dorn91-1. Accessed on: 4.7.2018.

Espin J, Schlander M, Godman B, Anderson P, Mestre-Ferrandiz J, Borget I. Hutchings A, Flostrand S, Parnaby A, Jommi C. (2018) Projecting pharmaceutical expenditure in EU5 to 2021: Adjusting for the impact of discounts and rebates. *Applied Health Economics and Health Policy* 16(6):803–817.

Ess SM, Schneeweiss S, Szucs TD. (2003) European healthcare policies for controlling for drug expenditure. *PharmacoEconomics* 21(2):89–103.

European PPP Expertise Center (EPEC). (2017) Market Update Review of the European PPP Market in 2017. www.eib.org/attachments/epec/epec_market_update_2017_en.pdf. Accessed on: 4.8.2019.

Ferrario A, Kanavos P. (2015). Dealing with uncertainty and high prices of new medicines: A comparative analysis of the use of managed entry agreements in Belgium, England, the Netherlands and Sweden. *Social Science & Medicine* 124:39–47.

Forster SP, Stegmaier J, Spycher R, Seeger S. (2014) Virtual pharmaceutical companies: Collaborating flexibly in pharmaceutical development. *Drug Discovery Today* 19(3):348–355.

Gemmill MC, Thomson S, Mossialos E. (2008) What impact do prescription drug charges have on efficiency and equity? Evidence from high-income countries. *International Journal for Equity in Health* 7. https://doi.org/10.1186/1475-9276-7-12.

Gereffi G. (1983) *Pharmaceutical Industry and Dependency in the Third World.* Princeton University Press: Princeton, NJ, USA, p. 223.

Greer SL, Bekker M, de Leeuw E, Wismar M. Helderman JK, Ribeiro S, Stuckler D (2017) Policy, politics and public health. *European Journal of Public Health* 27(4):40–43.

Griffiths P, Vingoe L, Hunt N, Mounteney J, Hartnoll R. (2000) Drug information systems, early warning, and new drug trends: Can drug monitoring systems become more sensitive to emerging trends in drug consumption? *Subsistence Use & Misuse* 35(6–8):811–844.

Gundgaard J. (2005) Income related inequality in prescription drugs in Denmark. *Pharmacoepidemiology and Drug Safety* 14(5):307–317.

Holloway KA, Henry D. (2014) WHO Essential medicines policies and use in developing and transitional countries: An analysis of reported policy implementation and medicines use surveys. *PLoS Med* 11(9): e1001724.

Hone T, Gurol-Urganci I, Millett C, Başara B, Akdağ R, Atun R. (2017) Effect of primary health care reforms in Turkey on health service utilization and user satisfaction. *Health Policy and Planning* 32(1):57–67.

King DR, Kanavos P. (2002) Encouraging the use of generic medicines: Implications for transition economies. *Croatian Medical Journal* 43(4):462–469.

Kockaya G, Yenilmez FB, Sharaf A, Ammar H. (2017) Increasing trend on Turkish un-licenced medicine market: A general overview analysis. *Value in Health* 20(9):A668–A669.

Kumru S, Top M. (2018) Pricing and reimbursement of generic pharmaceuticals in Turkey: Evaluation of hypertension drugs from 2007 to 2013. *Health Policy and Technology* 7(2):182–193.

Kyle MK. (2007) Pharmaceutical price controls and entry strategies. *Review of Economics and Statistics* 89(1):88–99.

Lambrelli D, O'Donnell O. (2011) The impotence of price controls: Failed attempts to constrain pharmaceutical expenditures in Greece. *Health Policy* 101(2):162–171.

Laverty H, Gunn M, Goldman M. (2012) Improving R&D productivity of pharmaceutical companies through public–private partnership: Experiences from the Innovative Medicines Initiative. *Expert Review of PharmacoEconomics & Outcomes Research* 12(5):545–548.

Lichtenberg FR, Tatar M, Caliskan Z. (2017) The impact of pharmaceutical innovation on health outcomes and utilization in Turkey: A re-examination. *Health Policy and Technology* 6(2):226–233.

Ministry of Finance (MoF). (2017). Budget Realization Report (Bumko). www.bumko.gov.tr/Eklenti/10835,2017mybutcebeklentileriraporupdf.pdf?0. Accessed on: 4.4.2019.

Ministry of Health (MoH) Health Statistics Year Book. (2015) General Directorate of Health Research. Ankara. Turkey. https://dosyasb.saglik.gov.tr/Eklenti/23530,2015-yili29pdf.pdf?0. Accessed on: 22.2.2019.

Moon S, Jambert E, Childs M, von Schoen-Angerer T. (2011) A win-win solution? A critical analysis of tiered pricing to improve access to medicines in developing countries. *Globalization and Health* 7(39):1–11.

O'Donnell O, van Doorslaer E, Wagstaff A, Lindelow M. (2008) *Analyzing health equity using household survey data. A Guide to Techniques and Their Implementation.* The World Bank: Washington, D.C.

Organization for Economic Co-operation and Development (OECD). (2017) Indicators Health at a Glance 2017. www.oecd-ilibrary.org/docserver/health_glance-2017en.pdf?expires=1550642130&id=id&accname=ocid43023557&checksum=11DB1EFB340DE496AE54E08239F6CAC3. Accessed on: 4.8.2019.

Osei-Kyei R, Chan APC. (2015) Review of studies on the critical success factors for Public–Private Partnership (PPP) projects from 1990 to 2013. *International Journal of Project Management* 33(6):1335–1346.

Pejcic AV, Jakovljevic M. (2017) Pharmaceutical expenditure dynamics in the Balkan countries. *Journal of Medical Economics* 20(10):1013–1017.

Pérez-Casas C, Herranz E, Ford N. (2001) Pricing of drugs and donations: Options for sustainable equity pricing. *Tropical Medicine & International Health* 6(11):960–964.

Pezzola A, Sweet CM. (2016) Global pharmaceutical regulation: The challenge of integration for developing states. *Globalization and Health* 12(85):1–18.

PPP Market in 2017. www.eib.org/attachments/epec/epec_market_update_2017_en.pdf. 1–11. Accessed on: 4.9.2019.

Raymond H, Chui M. (2009) The pharmemerging future. *Pharmaceutical Executive* 29(7):44.

Reich MR. (1995) The politics of health sector reform in developing countries: Three cases of pharmaceutical policy. *Health Policy* 32(1–3):47–77.

Rodrik D. (2018) Populism and the economics of globalization. *Journal of International Business Policy* 1:12–33.

Scherer FM. (2001) The link between gross profitability and pharmaceutical R&D spending. *Health Affairs* (Millwood) 20(5):216–220.

Sirgy MJ, Lee DJ, Yu GB. (2011) Consumer sovereignty in healthcare: Fact or fiction? *Journal of Business Ethics* 101:459–474.

Social Security Institution (SSI). (2019) Health Statistics Database. Retrieved from: www.sgk.gov.tr/wps/portal/kurumsal/istatistikler. Accessed on: 21.2.2019.

Stuckler D. (2017) The dispossessed: A public health response to the rise of the far-right in Europe and North America. *The European Journal of Public Health* 27(1):5–6.

Tatar M. Ozgen H, Sahin B, Belli P, Berman P. (2007) Informal payments in the health sector: A case study from Turkey. *Health Affairs* (Millwood) 26(4):1029–1039.

Tengilimoglu D, Kısa A, Ekiyor A. (2005) The pharmaceutical sales rep/physician relationship in Turkey. *Health Marketing Quarterly* 22(1):21–39.

Toklu HZ, Dulger GA, Hıdıroglu S, Akici A, Yetim A, Gannemoglu HM, Gunes H. (2012) Knowledge and attitudes of the pharmacists, prescribers and patients towards generic drug use in Istanbul – Turkey. *Pharma Practice* (Granada) 10(4):199–206.

Tooole AA. (2012) The impact of public basic research on industrial innovation: Evidence from the pharmaceutical industry. *Research Policy* 41(1):1–12.

Top M, Sungur C. (2018) Opinions and evaluations of stakeholders in the implementation of the public-private partnership (PPP) model in integrated health campuses (city hospitals) in Turkey. *International Journal of Health Policy and Planning* 34(1):e241–e263.

Vural I. (2015) Politics, reforms, and regulation of pharma prices and expenditures in Turkey over the 2000s. In Pharmaceutical Prices in the 21st Century. Zaheer-Ud-Din Babar (ed.) (pp. 267–295), Springer International: Cham, p. 289.

Vural I. (2017) Financialization in health care: An analysis of private equity fund investments in Turkey. *Social Science & Medicine* 187:276–286.

World Health Organization (WHO). 2015. WHO Guideline on Country Pharmaceutical Pricing Policies. https://apps.who.int/iris/bitstream/handle/10665/153920/9789241549035_eng.pdf?sequence=1. Accessed on: 20.4.2019.

Yılmaz ES, Kockaya G, Yenilmez FB, Saylan M., Tatar M, Akbulat A, Gursoz H, Kerman S. (2016) Impact of health policy changes on trends in the pharmaceutical market in Turkey. *Value in Health Regional Issues* 10:48–52.

Yilmaz ES. (2016) Impact of health policy changes on trends in the pharmaceutical market in Turkey. *Value in Health Regional Issues* 10:48–52.

Index

For Product Safety Concerns and Information please contact our EU
representative GPSR@taylorandfrancis.com
Taylor & Francis Verlag GmbH, Kaufingerstraße 24, 80331 München, Germany